WLM228

By the same author

Psychotherapy: A personal approach
Illusion and Reality: The meaning of anxiety
The Origins of Unhappiness
How to Survive without Psychotherapy

Taking Care
An Alternative to Therapy

David Smail

CONSTABLE · LONDON

First published in Great Britain 1987
by J.M.Dent & Sons Ltd
This paperback edition first published 1998
by Constable and Company Limited
3 The Lanchesters, 162 Fulham Palace Road
London W6 9ER
Copyright © David Smail 1987
Reprinted 1999
ISBN 0 09 477420 X
The right of David Smail to be identified as the
author of this work has been asserted by him in
accordance with the Copyright, Designs and Patents Act 1988
Printed in Great Britain by
St Edmundsbury Press Ltd, Bury St Edmunds, Suffolk

A CIP catalogue record for this book
is available from the British Library

Contents

To the memory of Don Bannister

New Preface

Of all my written works, *Taking Care* provides the clearest statement of issues concerning psychotherapy and society which I have been struggling with all my professional life. Less ambiguously than previous books (*Psychotherapy: A personal approach; Illusion and Reality*), it sets out what I see as the limitations of conventional approaches to psychotherapy. At the same time, it lays the ground for subsequent works (*The Origins of Unhappiness; How to Survive without Psychotherapy*) to elaborate, respectively, a detailed theoretical analysis of psychological distress and a kind of manual for 'ordinary people' to understand the significance of their own suffering.

Principally because, in my view, it became a victim of publishing take-overs in the eighties, *Taking Care* was not as widely read as its predecessor, *Illusion and Reality*. I have always regretted this: for me, it is the profounder and more mature of the two. I am therefore particularly grateful to Carol O'Brien and Constable for bringing it out in this edition.

It is, to put it mildly, a bracing read, bucking the trends of fashion, I have to admit, almost foolhardily. For the most part, works of popular psychology – and many academic approaches too, come to that – seek to reassure their audience that all is not as bad as it seems and that their ills can be overcome through the exercise of some kind of technique or other discovered, or at least propounded, by the author. Such, I think, is the secret of the success of much of the best-selling literature in the psychology and psychotherapy field: it feeds on the hopes and fantasies of people struggling against very difficult odds and only too ready to jump at relatively painless solutions.

No such Panglossian philosophy underlies this work, I fear. Reading it ten years on, even I was slightly taken aback in places at the bleakness of the view of society it portrays. The message is that, far from things being not as bad as they seem, they are in fact worse, and the (largely commercial) apparatus of social control through which the relatively more powerful maintain their advantage over the relatively less powerful has become perfected to the point where it is virtually insuperable. So far as *repairing* the damage done by this society is concerned, psychotherapy is an irrelevance: at best it is a temporary comfort, at worst a distraction. There is no substitute for taking care, and in the long run how a society takes care of its members is a political, not a therapeutic matter.

Uncompromising though this message undoubtedly is, I do not regret it, and indeed I have since retracted no part of it. And although it is stated in these pages with some ferocity, in places, it carries with it a level of reassurance for those in psychological pain more profound than that provided by any form of 'treatment'. For the whole point is that emotional suffering of the kind which comes to be labelled 'neurotic' or 'clinical' is the result not of the individual's inadequacies, shortcomings, personal or genetic weaknesses, but of the *inescapable* infliction on vulnerable bodies of noxious social influences which have their origin, most often, far beyond the orbit of our personal lives.

The issues of responsibility and blame, of what we can and cannot will (spelt out in most detail, perhaps, in *How to Survive without Psychotherapy*), constitute a theme which recurs throughout my written work, and though I have been hammering away at it in one form or another for twenty years, it is still, I think, the one most people find hardest to grasp. The core of our problem is stated about as clearly as I can manage in Chapter Four, where I try to show that it is the apparent indubitability of our personal experience – our intimate knowledge of our feelings – which makes it so difficult for us to conceive of the source of our difficulties as *outside* ourselves. We *feel* it inside, so we think that that is where it must indeed originate, and we are, therefore, easily persuaded that it is *we* who are responsible for what ails us.

We give up this notion, if at all, only with the greatest reluctance, for we feel that to do so robs us of our freedom and our agency. In my subsequent writing I have tried to elaborate the point that we do have freedom and agency, but only to the extent that they are *accorded to* us. The power(s) to choose and to act are not God-given, personal attributes, simply matters of 'will-power', but social acquisitions dependent on the availability of essentially material resources in the world outside our skins. Though some may find it paradoxical, I resolutely maintain that this is, for those who are suffering, a counsel not of despair, but of comfort. Certainly, in my work as a clinical psychologist, I have met many people who have found it comforting; better to be suffering than to be sub-standard.

This book is, therefore, more a critique of the society which gives rise to psychological distress than of the approaches to therapy which have been spawned to assuage it; the focus has shifted from individual experience (as in *Illusion and Reality*) to social structure.

It was not difficult to see ten years ago how pervasive make-believe and wishfulness were becoming as ways of interpreting experience and constructing means of social control – I claim no prophetic powers – but even so the true prophets of 'postmodernity' (Jean-François Lyotard, Jean Baudrillard) may have seemed to be over-stating their case. Where I wrote in Chapter One of our failure to distinguish between emdodied reality and dream-like imagery, the representation of war as an aesthetic, electronic experience was still almost five years off. The nineties, however have seen the extension of imagery and make-believe right into the core of the body politic and the threats to our embodied hold on reality which were identified in the earlier chapters of this book are now represented within the official institutions of our society more as a virtue than a nightmare.

The further disintegration of any idea that politics could be the proper concern of the citizenry is particularly to be deplored. In what has become a kind of apolitical, almost 'virtual' government, issues affecting the material reality of our lives, along with concepts of economic fairness and social justice, have been set aside in favour of, for example, variants on the theme of 'responsibility'. Rather than either the regulation or the overt exercise of oppressive power, there is an attempt to maintain control (whether of scapegoats, such as the teachers, or of corrupt commercial institutions selling pension plans) through shaming and admonishment. The manipulation of image, the frank abandonment of actuality for appearance (for example the celebration of fashion as an 'industry') have become not just ideological tools of government but the very process of government itself. Government has thus become the management of appearance; what is done to people is considered indistinguishable from what they think has been done to them (hence the successful politician's obsession with 'focus groups' and the consequent inevitability of demagoguery); magic is officially rehabilitated at every cultural level – science and soothsaying are seen as but alternative ways to 'the truth'. The collapse of the distinction between public and private which so concerns me in these pages is now virtually complete.

And yet, of course, reality will not be gainsaid. We are still embodied creatures in a real world even though the concept of a 'real world' has been hopelessly undermined by market rhetoric. What has happened, of course, is that the demands of global Business have put out of sight and beyond the reach of our criticism – beyond, most significantly, the power of national governments to control – the actual levers of power which constistute the ultimate influences on our lives. A 'Labour' Prime Minister can smugly extol the virtues of a 'flexible labour market' because the 'reality' of his world does not include being able to influence the policies of huge multi-national companies – he can only dance to their tune. And for the men and women thrown out of work in the interests of 'flexibility' there are no officially authorized words with which to criticize their condition; if their distress is not simply dumb, it can be given form only in the language of personal responsibility and inadequacy. The unemployed are 'jobseekers' or 'welfare-dependants' and rather than being able to earn the means of their livelihood they are offered either moral exhortation or counselling.

We need more than ever before to rescue the reality of our world, if only because of the pain which is inflicted on the lives of so many 'ordinary' people. Our virtual reality is bought at too high a price. Even in relatively prosperous Britain the suffering of those at the bottom of the heap – and they are no small minority – is a social outrage. Though not exactly a secret (ask any inner-city teacher or health worker) the extent of this suffering is resolutely obscured by the official institutions of society, not least the therapy and counselling industry. The very first thing we have to do, therefore, is to establish with fearless clarity what the nature of our predicament is, and that may indeed prove a somewhat harrowing process. Our real problem, however, is in knowing where to go from there.

It is easy enough to construct formulae for how our personal lives should be lived – the philosophy of life sketched in Chapter Seven, for example, still seems to me a fair enough ideal – but turning insight into action is not simply a matter of the exercise of personal will, for as individuals we are not in control of what we do. In this book I make the case for taking care rather than providing therapy, but *how* that is to be achieved requires a political analysis and understanding beyond the scope of these pages. One thing, however, is certain: it will require the exercise of social power.

David Smail
Nottingham, 1997

Introduction

Our accustomed ways of looking at the world suggest that we all live in an unalterable, shared reality which exists quite independently of any feelings we might have about how it *ought* to be. Equally, our accustomed view of knowledge – especially scientific knowledge – is that it gives a dispassionate, disinterested description of the way things *are*, again independently of how we might like them to be.

These accustomed ways of looking at the world and viewing knowledge have long been known – at least by many of those whose business it is to think about such things – to be false.

In fact, the 'reality' we believe in is an illusion. In fact, our 'dispassionate' knowledge is highly partial and selective: it has aims and purposes inextricable from the *interests* of power. We use knowledge to subordinate nature, and that includes ourselves.

These issues may seem a long way from the concerns of a psychologist whose job it is to try to understand and if possible alleviate the emotional distress of individual people. However, having worked for a number of years in the field of psychological 'treatment', I have become convinced, in the first place, that these issues are central to an understanding of human despair, and in the second that they should no longer remain the particular property of 'those whose business it is to think about such things'. These issues are everybody's concern, and though it may be in the professional interest to limit serious consideration of them to the experts, to do so would not be, and is not, for the public good.

The central argument of this book is a very simple one, but, obscured by my professional blinkers, it has taken me nearly three decades to see it: psychological distress occurs for reasons which make it incurable by therapy, but which are certainly not beyond the powers of human beings to influence. We suffer pain because we do damage to each other, and we shall continue to suffer pain as long as we continue to do the damage. The way to alleviate and mitigate distress is for us *to take care of* the world and the other people in it, not to *treat* them.

Although (to me, but I am sure also to many others) this 'insight' has now become blindingly obvious, it is extraordinarily difficult to marshall the arguments and evidence which support it, since they so often run counter to our customary ways of seeing and thinking about things. It is, however, my belief that one cannot expect people to give up the hope (not to mention the resources)

1

they invest in 'treatment' until they have gained access to and had a chance to consider for themselves what the arguments and evidence are. And one cannot expect the sum of human distress to diminish until we give up our investment in treatment, and address instead the daunting task of taking care.

In my previous book, *Illusion and Reality: The Meaning of Anxiety,** my basic concerns were not different from those informing the present work, but my focus was particularly upon individuals and their experience of anxiety within the compass of their own lives. My aim was to try to offer encouragement to people (that is, all of us) who have been bludgeoned out of their understanding of the world by a remorseless 'objectivity', to risk trusting themselves to become the 'subjects' that, in fearful secret, they somehow know themselves to be. This time my focus is wider; having, as it were, stated the dilemma in terms of the way it presents itself in our immediate experience, I want now to broaden the view to show how that experience is formed and influenced by the social and cultural structures which we inhabit, and to suggest what the implications of that may be for the way we should conduct ourselves towards one another.

An attempt to understand the influence of social and cultural structures takes one beyond present times and places, and challenges familiar and unthinkingly accepted views of what 'society' is about. In the following pages I shall suggest a number of things which may well seem at first – or even second – sight hard to swallow: for example, that the world we seem to know, and which seems so unalterably hard, and real and resistant to our will, is in several important ways the illusory creation of our wishes, the fabrication of our dreams. Indeed, there is a sense in which dreaming, even when awake, is *inescapable*. We are, as it were, doomed to 'grasp' reality only through our *interpretation* of it, and hence we cannot really grasp it at all. But we *can*, as I shall also argue, have *respect* for it: we may dream recklessly, or we may go carefully because we know we are dreaming.

Again, I shall argue that what we take to be dispassionate knowledge is in fact suffused with *interest*; that is, our knowledge is inseparable from the uses to which we wish to put it – we *exploit* our knowledge in order to *exploit* the world's resources (including people), and because so much of that exploitation is fundamentally dishonourable, we hide its nature from ourselves (we 'repress' it). My particular concern here will of course be with psychological knowledge, and again I shall have the difficult – and to many people perhaps unpalatable – task of suggesting that the main

*Dent, 1984.

2

use to which psychological knowledge has been put has been the exploitation of some people by others for purposes which, though they do not appear in those others' conscious awareness, nevertheless suit them rather well.

Furthermore, if one is to understand the workings of interest, particularly in relation to psychology and 'treatment', one must investigate the sources of the plausibility in which it manages to clothe itself. In part, I believe, these are to be traced to an age-old and ever-present attraction to magic (which also shapes much of our dreaming). Magic, indeed, is not at all a relic of the past, but is found at the very kernel of our enthusiasm for science.

These factors (our wishful dreaming, magic, and interest) combine with what we take to be the point of our lives – the 'pursuit of happiness' – to enslave us within a society in which exploitation and indifference are the norm. In this society also, the intellectual and conceptual means whereby we might get a purchase on our predicament are largely obscured from us. Nowhere is this more so than in the case of psychological distress and its treatment, in which our ideas about why we suffer as we do, and whom we are to 'blame', as well as how we may change or be 'cured', are shaped by our social and cultural concerns much more to justify and permit further exploitation than to allow us an insight into the true reasons for our ills.

Far from being repairable machines, human beings are embodied organisms on whom damage will at best always leave a scar. We simply cannot get away with using and abusing each other as we do, and it is small wonder that the ways of life into which we have uncritically fallen, and which we take for granted as the natural response to an inescapable reality, reverberate so disastrously in our conduct towards and experience of each other – that is, in our 'relationships', where, again without noticing, we have carried exploitation to the very heart of our social undertakings, placing it between man and woman, and parent and child.

The sense of 'therapy' which the subtitle of this book calls into question is that in which therapy is 'officially' offered (and undoubtedly widely accepted in the public mind) as a *technical* procedure for the cure or adjustment of emotional or psychological 'disorder' in individual people. There are 'unofficial' aspects of psychotherapy – recognized at least implicitly by many of its practitioners – which I would not want to question, and indeed in pursuance of which this book could be said to be written. These aspects, however, are, in contrast with the grandiose claims and aspirations of most 'schools' of psychotherapy, extremely limited (sadly necessary palliatives in a disordered society) and not justifiably professionally 'patentable'. Elaboration of them should in no

3

way distract us from the much more essential task of trying to understand and prevent the processes whereby we come to inflict upon each other so much incurable damage.

As a matter of fact, though their stated profession and unstated interest may be to offer cure, most therapists of good will also play an inadvertently subversive role within the society which damages us so profoundly. As I tried to show in *Psychotherapy: A Personal Approach*,* what most often psychotherapists *actually* (as opposed to professedly) do, is to *negotiate* a view of what the patient's predicament is about which both patient and therapist can agree (which is to establish, as closely as one ever can, what is the truth of the matter), and then to *encourage* the patient to do what he or she can to confront those elements of the predicament which admit of some possibility of alteration. This almost inevitably means that patients begin to criticize aspects of a social 'reality' which before they had always taken for granted, and, with courage or grace, to learn actively to dissent from and oppose the constraints it had placed upon them: to overcome the tyranny of objectivity. I would now lay more emphasis than I did in that book on the value of *comfort*: for many people, psychotherapy provides the only source of comfort they are likely to find in what has been, for them at least, a predominantly cruel world.

The *actual* possible achievements of therapy may thus be summarized very briefly as establishing what is the case ('demystification'), and providing comfort and encouragement. Inasmuch as this book is addressed primarily to people trying to make sense of their own and others' distress, it is my hope that lessons I have learned from the experience of psychotherapy (as I have come to understand it) may to some extent transfer to these pages.

The process of demystification, the examination and clearing of the confusions which surround the person's deceived or self-deceiving view of what lies behind the 'symptoms', often forms the longest part of the therapeutic enterprise. There are, it is true, therapists who feel that, as long as *they* are sure of how they can make patients confront the difficulties which beset them, there is really no point in spending much time in demystification: what matters, they say, is getting on with tackling the problems, not investigating the reasons why they arose in the first place. I do not myself agree with this view, though I have no doubt that it may sometimes 'work'. It seems to me essential for people to enter into, to have the full opportunity to alter and argue with the processes whereby someone else arrives at a formulation of 'the problem'; the alternative constitutes reliance upon an authoritarian or

*Dent, 1978.

4

'parentalist' elite which in the long run infantilizes and makes dependent – embodies, indeed, a form of tyranny.

It is of course not possible in a book to enter into a dialogue with the reader, and hence the *negotiative* element of attempts at 'demystification' has to be missing. I shall, then, have to rely upon arguments which I hope will persuade, and forego the opportunity of *listening* which is so essential to reaching an understanding. Nobody, I am sure, who is fundamentally antipathetic to any particular view is persuaded of its truth by argument. I shall, therefore, be preaching to the at least half converted; in any case I believe that the most a writer can hope for is to illuminate and articulate ideas and views which are already partially formed in the reader.

It is then in a *kind* of demystification process that the first six chapters of this book (those, that is, whose contents have been briefly sketched above) are intended to be engaged. The intention is to suggest that our ordinary ways of considering our lives and 'relationships' (i.e. the other people in them) obscure a view of how corrupt, exploitative and emotionally impoverished and damaging our social organization, and hence our conduct towards each other, have become. In the course of making my argument I cannot rely on cast-iron 'evidence', but will have to trust to the all-too-fallible methods of persuasion (as for example occasional reference to what may turn out to be entirely idiosyncratic elements of my own experience) by which I may hope to strike in the reader a sympathetic chord. Some of the arguments I shall marshall are based on ideas I know I have gleaned from others, and some, no doubt, on ideas which I have forgotten that I have gleaned from others. Whatever their source, all of them are ideas which illuminate and make sense of my experience during the conduct of psychotherapy: they clarify, for me anyway, the nature of distress.

The final two chapters are written in the hope that some *encouragement* may be derived from them. There are in fact no magic answers to our predicament, no dreaming away of our real, embodied, presence in the world. There is no escape from the necessity to give up an infantile longing for blissful ease, to grow to maturity and to take care both of our environment and of each other. We have to rediscover a morality which is not moralistic, and construct a society which both acknowledges and makes what provision it can for the *difficulties* involved in creating tolerance, forbearance, justice and care. We talk a lot about love, but (as I suggested in *Illusion and Reality*) there is not a great deal of it about. We cannot, therefore, simply love each other better; we have first to make a society in which love may take root and thrive.

I cannot claim to be optimistic about the prospects of attaining any such society (could anyone, who sees the lack of restraint in our history and the destructive intent of our technology?), but it might, with the very greatest effort, just be possible.

There is probably not very much of *comfort* in all this. However, my experience both personally and professionally is that the greatest comfort derives from having one's view, however despairing it may be, confirmed by someone else who is not afraid to share it. As long, then, as this book helps some people in their quest to identify the roots of their unease, I hope it may even be comforting. It would certainly comfort me to think that here or there it might find an echo.

There is one central and essential point I wish to emphasize above all others in this introduction, and to beg the reader to bear in mind throughout what follows: it is neither my wish nor my intention to engender in him or her any sense of guilt or blame. It is extremely difficult, perhaps impossible, seriously to criticize our society and our conduct toward each other without challenging very fundamental and widely shared assumptions, without showing anger and having at times almost deliberately to shock. Even the most constructive criticism, if it is to avoid superficiality, necessitates seeing some very familiar things in some very unfamiliar ways. There are thus some elements of trying to 'negotiate' a view which just cannot be at all times measured and reasonable and cool. But it is part of the very heart of my argument that no body – singular or collective – is to *blame* for the predicament in which we find ourselves. We are all, certainly, *responsible*, in the sense that nobody but we ourselves wreak on each other the havoc we do, but the concept of blame is one which mystifies and obscures the processes whereby this comes about. (Blame is an effective means of manipulating people and groups, not a valid concept for understanding them.) As anyone who has an intimate concern with human misery knows, blame and guilt, invoked as explanations, are simply ways of evading the difficulties involved in tackling it. The same, it seems to me, is likely to be true of misery on a societal scale.

1
Dreaming and Wishing: The Individual and Society

'All life is a dream, and dreams are just dreams.'

What seemed to me as a schoolboy no more than a poetic affectation useful for quoting in exams, comes to mind thirty years later as a statement of the simple truth.

Perhaps all that signifies is that literature is wasted on some schoolboys; perhaps anyway Calderón* meant something entirely different by his words from what I now understand by them. However that may be, it seems to me that we may be sunk more deeply into our dreams than at any previous time in our recorded history, and in any case more deeply than we can afford to be, for our dreams are full of a destructive rage and hatred, a frustrated craving for omnipotence, a desperation for satisfaction beyond the bounds of mere greed, through which we may dream ourselves to our own annihilation.

We can see the world only in the ways that human beings, with their own particular ways of sensing and experiencing (and *interpreting* sensation and experience) *can* see it. Whatever reality there may be beyond the 'reality' which filters to us through our individual, historical and cultural ways of seeing, we shall never be able to say what it 'is'. We have, of course, a naive belief in a scientifically establishable, objective reality, but subscribing to that belief is in truth doing no more than taking, in a very grandiose way, what is merely our best guess so far about the nature of things *as* the nature of things. We have yet fully to accept that we can *never* get beyond guesswork.

So we are dreamers within a reality we cannot ever completely know, but which is nevertheless vulnerable to our conduct. Our lives are dreamt within a world, indeed a universe, which *permits* our dreaming and exists independently of it. Though we cannot know our world, we can certainly dream its destruction (and thereby put an end also to our dreaming).

That 'primitive man' lives in a dream is easy enough for most of us to grasp as we read of his nervous transactions with a world of ghostly ancestry and dangerous magic. What we find less easy to see is that our own world is to just about the same extent constructed out of superstitious fantasies, centring, in our case,

*In his play *Life Is a Dream*, 1635.

mainly around images of conquest and wealth. Furthermore, our naive belief in a scientifically establishable objective reality renders us dangerously blind to the influence of our dreaming. Less wise than the Australian Aborgines, we do not acknowledge our origin in a 'dream time', and have not traced its contribution to our 'scientifically established reality'. We mistakenly trust our reality, therefore, not to be affected by 'primitive' dreaming: we are not sufficiently on our guard against the influence of our dreams.

Dreams vary in the degree of their 'primitiveness', but this is to be judged more by the extent to which they are infused by wishful self-concern than by any lack of correspondence they may have with what we assume to be 'objective reality'.

Human beings are, so to speak, engines of symbolism. We turn the reality we cannot finally know into a kind of endlessly enriching compost of symbols, of which our wide-awake, conscious words are only one, and by no means necessarily the most profound, aspect. Anyone who has 'watched' his or her thoughts (i.e. self-addressed speech) turn at the point of sleep into 'pictures' cannot fail to be astounded by the economy, complexity and beauty of the process of symbolic transformation. Since it tends not to have words attached to it, and since we find it very hard to 'remember' without the use of language, this process is an extremely difficult one to capture. Although I know I have experienced it quite frequently, I can only think of a couple of examples.

Sitting in a London underground train, for instance, I watch the cables writhe past along the tunnel wall. Some are thicker than others; they run neatly parallel, until suddenly they switch position, cross over, alter their height, branch unexpectedly, swerve a little. I just catch myself 'realizing' that the cables 'are' an argument; they are a complex logical discourse; in some absolutely *direct* way they display the nature of an intellectual thesis. Again, one hot afternoon, I look slightly sleepily out of the window down at the car park outside. Suddenly the car park – the arrangement of the cars, their colours, the way the sunlight reflects off them – is absolutely *full of meaning* (I cannot say what, for I am surprised into wakefulness and have no time to put words to the meaning before it has gone).

I suspect that our world – the world, that is, of 'developed' Western civilization – is as saturated with our dream-meanings as are the cave walls of any Stone Age hunters. We live with the world we cannot know (in the way we think we would like to) in a relation of symbolic reciprocity. We extract from the world meanings and metaphors which we then project back into it as objective characteristics, though of course there is nothing truly objective about them.

At any moment, waking or sleeping, experience reaches us through an accretion of meaning, all of it to *some* extent individually and culturally idiosyncratic, which has, as it were, become wired into our bodies from previous experience. This accretion of meaning thus gives form and colour to everything we experience in the present, providing a kind of symbolic background to what we take to be reality. In this sense, we dream all the time. Perhaps the underground cables have more in common with the caveman's bison than we might suspect.* More than just dreaming inside our own heads, we dream *into* as well as *out of* the world: our psychological relation to the world is one of continuous symbolic interchange. The depth, complexity and significance of that relation is quite awe-inspiring; symbolization of this kind, asleep or awake, is the very opposite of primitive. There is no shame in our being dreamers.

'All life is a dream', if true, seemed to my schoolboy self a potential reason for taking life less seriously than otherwise one might. However, the reverse now seems to me the case. If I dream you, and you dream me (and, of course, we *do:* how else explain the rapid shifts in perception of each other we undergo, the discovery in time that we are more separate than we thought, that wife is not mother, husband not knight?), then how careful we must be with each other. For if all there is for us is dreaming there is no possibility of waking to find that the harm we have done each other was *just* a dream. Over and over again, as a species, we 'awake' from our dreams to find our hands covered in blood.

There are all kinds of dreaming, and it is important not to get carried away by the metaphor of 'life as a dream' to the point where we lose a conception of reality. Even though we cannot directly know reality as something 'in itself', existing quite objectively apart from our symbolic understanding of it, we can attempt to 'unwind' it as far as possible from our wishful fantasies.

This, no doubt, is what science, at its best, achieves. But all too quickly science itself becomes enmeshed in our autistic reveries of power, so that we use it as a vehicle for our covert aims and borrow its authority to justify our ravaging of the world and each other.

The wishful fantasies we dream in our beds at night – the kind of which Freud began, at least, to articulate an understanding – present no great problem of themselves. (In fact, they need no articulate understanding since their whole meaning is *in*articulate

---

*This line of thought is pursued with great, if at times rather oppressive erudition by Susanne Langer in her three-volume *Mind: An Essay on Human Feeling*, Johns Hopkins University Press, 1967–82.

and in most respects quite sufficient unto itself.) As we sleep, we may fantasize any kind of satisfaction or horror with no more ill-effect than, perhaps, a slight feeling of unease or embarrassment for half the following day. But, awake, only a faithful respect for the unknowable reality of the world and the other people in it will prevent our enacting our dreams in potentially catastrophic ways. For what else is the man who takes an automatic rifle to mow down the shoppers in an American supermarket doing but dreaming?

If we are to unwind ourselves from the strands of base magic which are so thickly interwoven in our dreams we need to remind ourselves that we are not simply pictures, or shadows, or images, but *bodies* in a *world*. In the second half of this century there has been an increasing awareness of the dangerous seductiveness of the image, though interpreted differently by different writers.* At times, even, it becomes unclear which is more important to us – the image or the actuality. In the political sphere particularly, though by no means solely, the explicit concern of the actors (some of them trained as such!) as well as the commentators is with the adequacy of their image, the effectiveness of the 'P.R.' battles which seek to present us with credibility as a higher value than truth. The awful danger, of course, is that enactment of the fantasies which such 'images' create can, and does, result in the mutilation of our bodies and our world.

Contributing to this state of affairs, no doubt, is the fact that our very experience of the world is becoming increasingly insubstantial and disconnected from any bodily involvement in it. For example, whether presenting 'fact' or 'fantasy', the television – on which most of us depend for any kind of understanding of world affairs – deals solely in images. It thus becomes increasingly difficult to differentiate the images of our dreaming sleep from those of our waking televisual experience, and gradually the laborious, uneditable nature of our bodily experience of the world seems to become

---

*Daniel Boorstin, for example, in *The Image* (Penguin Books, 1963) simply bemoans the usurpation by vulgar and synthetic imitativeness of values once the hallowed property of an appreciative elite. His thesis that the populace *demands* the trash supplied to it by an almost reluctant commercial world is absurd, though his exposure of the nature of the trash itself is brilliant. Guy Debord's *Society of the Spectacle* (Black and Red, 1983), born of the Paris riots in 1968, makes an altogether more plausible link between image and interest, though with great Gallic opacity. Most compelling of all is Christopher Lasch's *The Minimal Self* (Picador, 1985) in which the depths of our confusion between reality and illusion, and its dangers, are described with considerable power.

a kind of irksome, obsolete burden. Our dreams are so much more attractive, and it seems that technology makes them attainable.

At no time in our previous history can it have been so possible for people to 'experience' death and destruction – the actual death and destruction of real people – on such a wide scale but in such a disembodied and dislocated form. The danger is that we get so used to them in this form that we think we know what they're like and that they don't really hurt. Hence perhaps the numbed amazement written on the face of people who discover that 'it' has indeed 'happened to them'. Hence perhaps also the unhappy moral confusion and uncertainty surrounding the deaths of forty spectators at a televised football match – do we treat this as a real event demanding a flesh-and-blood response to the sensible agony of those involved, or do we sweep up the bodies like so many discarded cardboard containers of fried chicken and get on with the game? Our confusion is *genuine* – already our world is such that the values of embodied presence seem not necessarily to outweigh those of disembodied image.

And yet it is inconceivable that we shall ever be able to achieve what seems to be our covert aim – that is, to etherealize ourselves to the point where we become pure, disembodied images, as unencumbered as an electronic pulse. We are creatures of bone and tissue in a world upon which we depend for our bodily existence. If we persist in actually involving each other in the pursuit of our dream images, we shall discover that they are indeed dreams from which we cannot awake and that the sacrifices we make will be made not in pictures, but in tears and blood.

In our eagerness to escape the vulnerability to pain to which our nature as embodied beings exposes us, we construct a variety of technological and therapeutic 'solutions' which share a common origin in the wishful magic of dreaming. But no matter how hard we may try and how fervently we may believe in it, magic still does not work. The reluctant conclusion to which I have been driven after having worked for some years in the fields of psychology and psychotherapy – fields which are, as I shall argue later, deeply imbued with magic – is that human suffering arises from our embodied interaction with a world whose reality, though it cannot be known, cannot be wished away. A very significant part of the psychologist's role is continuous with that of the 'cunning man' and the astrologer, and as such is a sham. The evil that we do each other cannot be undone, at least not so easily as we like to think, and the ravages of the world cannot be erased.

Not for nothing, I believe, are so many people these days oppressed and frightened by a sense they have that 'things have got out of control', that people are the powerless victims of impersonal forces which are experienced as a strange and barely analysable mixture of malignity and inevitability — even necessity. It is as if these forces are uninfluenceable: we wait for them to crush us and to destroy our environment with the kind of hopeless resignation one imagines prisoners awaiting execution to feel.

Fifteen or so years ago, it was quite common for people who expressed a sense of impending doom, and who perhaps coupled this with some kind of untutored critique of the societal or technological influences they took to be responsible, to be diagnosed as mentally unstable in some way. I have several times in the past observed at first hand the label 'schizophrenic' being attached to someone on no better grounds than that they accounted for their emotional unease in terms judged by their psychiatrists to be 'pseudo-philosophical'. Nowadays, it seems, this sense of helplessness and threat has become much more general, and though the 'pseudo-philosophical' constructions of and reactions to it have become both more shared and more focused (e.g. in environmentalist movements and an upsurge of fundamentalist religious feeling) there are still many people who feel unable to formulate a clear idea of exactly what is wrong.

It is no longer plausible to suggest that people who feel this sort of unease are unstable or even mad (though this is a possibility that they themselves often consider with great trepidation). Our feelings seem rather to be indications of a social, not an individual, 'disease', and are to be taken absolutely seriously. 'Ordinary people', it seems, are swiftly becoming dislocated from any sense at all that they can influence or even identify those forces which shape their lives, and this both engenders a despair which is reflected in their relations with others and stimulates forms of defensiveness (such as denial, apathy, or ostrich-like optimism) which only serve to make things worse. The state of affairs, in any social community, in which people find themselves being carried along by forces which seem both destructive and out of reach of their influence, is a recipe for disaster.

'There have always been prophets of doom,' you may say, to which the answer must be that doom is prophesied only that it may be avoided. What I find much more chilling than prophecies of doom is the fact that doom has often enough already occurred with only one or two observers (out of millions) brave enough to say what they saw and to draw lessons for the future. The prophet of doom may indeed be an optimist alongside the observer of doom, who could under the circumstances scarcely be blamed for pessimism.

Take, for example, just one fragment of the experience of the psychoanalyst Wilfred Bion, who as a youth of barely twenty found himself blown into a shell-hole in a First World War battlefield, drenched in mud, water, and bits and pieces of other people's bodies – 'a kind of human soup'. It is surely not surprising that, having observed the 'progress' of humanity for the ensuing sixty years he should write:

> When the super clever monkeys with their super clever tools have blown themselves into a fit and proper state to provide delicate feeding for the coming lords and ladies of creation, super microbe sapiens, then the humans who cumber the earth will achieve their crowning glory, the gorgeous colours of putrescent flesh to rot and stink and cradle the new aristocracy.*

What is perhaps much more surprising is that so many people who have experienced similarly horrific circumstances to those Bion describes in his book, and so many of the rest of us who may in one way or another learn of them, continue, either by forgetting them, excusing them or even glorifying them, to believe in any future at all.

This may seem an unnecessarily drastic theme by which to illustrate our apparent inability to learn from our mistakes, and one far removed from the usual concerns of psychology. However, I make no apologies, since it seems to me that the everyday violence we do each other, the waste of human talent and squandering of human resources, the suspicion of and indifference toward each other which are such features of our alienated existence, all of which lead to a wreckage of human life which in its own way is quite bad enough, may eventually – perhaps quite soon – terminate in a frame of mind in which we really don't care if we try to destroy ourselves outright. This is not fanciful; it has happened before. The difference now is that 'we have the technology' to guarantee success.

Perhaps the most tragic aspect of human nature lies in its vulnerability to wishful magic. Perhaps, ultimately, it will prove to be its fatal aspect. Over and over again we abandon a rational intuition of our embodiment in a real world for passionate belief in alternative modes of existence in worlds created out of our imagination. Our genius as symbolizers and as users of language enables us to disregard the lessons of our bodily experience, and to construct acceptable versions of all our lowest motives and actions, in ways that, fortunately for them, are not available to less 'gifted' species, which are by contrast firmly anchored in an ineffable reality from which no flight of fancy can release them. A dead cat is a dead

*W. R. Bion *The Long Week-End*, Fleetwood Press, 1982.

cat, and could never become, for example, posthumous martyr to some warlike feline cause.

The cultural miasma that we have created inside our heads to preserve us from catching a glimpse of the mess we make of our world leads us also to be not easily moved by pity. If our response to physical pain and death is frequently uncertain, our awareness of frustration, deprivation and waste seems, on the face of things at least, largely absent, It was, for example, what he saw as the appalling waste of youth which inspired Paul Goodman to write a bitter critique* of American society of the fifties.

> In our society, bright lively children, with the potentiality for knowledge, noble ideals, honest effort, and some kind of worthwhile achievement, are transformed into useless and cynical bipeds, or decent young men trapped or early resigned, whether in or out of the organized system.

> In despair, the fifteen-year-olds hang around and do nothing at all, neither work nor play . . . They do not do their school work, for they are waiting to quit; and it is hard . . . for them to get part-time jobs. Indeed, the young fellows (not only delinquents) spend a vast amount of time doing nothing. They hang around together, but don't talk about anything, nor even — if you watch their faces — do they passively take in the scene. Conversely, at the movies, where the real scene is by-passed, they watch with absorbed fantasy, and afterward sometimes mimic what they saw.

It is sad that Goodman's book, apart from its forlorn thread of optimism more relevant today than ever, has not become a bible for anyone (i.e. all of us) who has responsibilities to the young. One wonders what Goodman would have made now of the dead-eyed hopelessness of so many young people whose only permissible aspiration is to acquire the plastic junk they appraise so listlessly in shopping-precinct windows, and one despairs that so passionate and articulate a warning should have gone so apparently unheeded.

No one is likely to become more aware of the extraordinary ingenuity possessed by human beings in the business of magically falsifying their experience than the psychotherapist. It is in the way we try to deal with the anguish arising from our existence in the world that one may see most clearly our reluctance to recognize its causes and get to grips effectively with its consequences. One of the earliest lessons learned by any moderately observant therapist is that what the patient says about his or her predicament is, for a

---

*P. Goodman, *Growing Up Absurd*, Vintage Books, 1956.

14

number of reasons (often outside the patient's knowledge or control), systematically distorted so as to hide its real significance. In fact, psychological malaise is the inevitable sequel of difficult or unfortunate aspects of the individual's relation to his or her world, but (conveniently for the person, society or both) is not recognized as such. To recognize the real reasons for psychological distress would, usually, be too painful or threatening, present difficulties too apparently insuperable, uncover hatred and recrimination too seemingly unbearable, reveal too much guilty subterfuge, or simply expose to view social injustice which would be too insupportable for the attendant difficulties to be kept within manageable bounds. Patients therefore magically interpret 'the problem' as something altogether more amenable to professional intervention; a lifetime of misery becomes an illness with a cure.

So far, psychotherapists, in seeing accurately enough that patients distort their experience so as to minimize the difficulties of its implications, have failed to realize that they themselves are playing a complementary part in this process of mystification by implicitly offering magic solutions for the 'problems' encountered. These are points upon which I shall expand in subsequent chapters, but what I want here to emphasize is that the therapeutic situation *as a whole* offers a rare insight into the way *collectively* we try to use magic to repair the damage we do to each other. Although it may be true that psychotherapists (and this was the abiding achievement of Freud and his colleagues) are able to remove some of the mystery from the individual person's anguish, they may end up only making matters worse if they set about trying to put things right merely through a process of, in the broadest sense, interpretation. We shall make, and in my view have made, no progress at all by *interpreting* human misery *merely* as the outcome of the individual's *mis*interpretation of his or her circumstances. What is so instructive about the therapeutic situation taken, again, as a whole, is that it shows clearly how we collude with each other in trying (on the patient's side) to falsify our experience and obscure our motives, and (on the therapist's) to offer magically painless ways out of the predicaments we create. A further instructive feature of the therapeutic situation, again one which I shall criticize in greater detail later, is that it seeks to understand and explain human distress precisely in *individual* terms, as well as implying that it may be 'cured' or ameliorated through efforts of individual consciousness.

For the moment, then, there are two lessons in particular from the experience of psychotherapy which I should wish to be borne clearly in mind. The first is that human beings easily misrepresent the reasons for their own anguish. The second is that those supposed to be most expert in the understanding of that anguish, being no more than human themselves, easily succeed in obscuring its nature even further. As a partial explanation of this I have concentrated so far upon our wishful fantasies, our greedy, magic-infused dreams. But at the centre of these is something altogether harder and more mundane: our interest.

Interest is the method in our madness, the force which pushes our dreams in some directions rather than others, the guilty secret which collectively we do our best to keep. It is by dragging interest into the open, I believe, that we shall most readily be able to understand the damage we do each other and the pain we cause. Not that in many ways interest is not perfectly manifest – indeed in these days in particular it shows itself in some of its aspects quite boldly – but still, of all our mystifications, the mystification of interest is the most developed and most defended at every level of society.

Among other (and more important) reasons for 'neurotic' self-deception is frequently to be found the individual's camouflaged interest – the rather base and shameful motive which is satisfied by the 'illness', the weakness, perhaps, which permits one person to tyrannize another. Indeed, almost any form of disability can be turned to the person's interest, and it is only the most unusual people who do not find *some* advantage to be gained from their lameness, deafness or blindness. However, our shameful weaknesses, if we are to put them to the fullest use, must be disguised, or, best, made unknown to ourselves, and for this the process of repression is most suitable: we *do* things, but we do not acknowledge (spell out in words) what we are doing. But this, and other reasons for 'neurotic' conduct identified as residing somehow within individuals, are not enough to explain their suffering. The operation of interest and repression at the individual level is useful mainly for offering us a clue to the understanding of their operation on an altogether wider scale.

In our everyday considerations of how societies work, repression is of course used in a rather different sense from that above. Groups or classes of people are repressed, it is thought, when the instruments of power are used quite consciously on the part of the ruling group or class to 'deal with' those it considers for one reason or another undesirable. And yet it is not only unhappy individuals who hide from themselves, by failing to acknowledge them, the operations whereby their interests are furthered. Through manipulation of the media of mass communication – the means whereby they spell out their intentions to their members – whole societies, and especially their governments, pursue the interests of those who wield power while claiming or appearing to pursue the welfare of all. In part this is of course quite conscious – few people these days, and least of all politicians, are unaware of the importance of 'image' – and yet, I suspect, most would feel (i.e. articulate to themselves) that the manipulation of image is aimed only at finding the 'best', most palatable way to present an entirely honourable policy. In fact, however, it is probably the case that societies no less than individuals successfully hide from themselves the dishonourable pursuit of their own interest by an exactly analogous process of not spelling it out. Furthermore, those people within a given society who threaten to discover the hidden interests and expose them to public criticism are likely to be repressed in *both* senses of the word: if they are not simply ignored or forgotten by public consciousness, they will be put down by power. They will be resisted just as bitterly as the psychoanalyst's interpretation of the individual patient's baser motives are resisted.

Nobody I know puts the issue of our interestedness with greater directness and simplicity than Leo Tolstoy. In a book (perhaps unsurprisingly in view of the nature of social repression) no longer widely read, nor indeed in print in Britain,* he suggests that the major cultural preoccupations of society have always been used in the service of the interests of the ruling group, covert vehicles for the unworthy motives of the powerful. First the Church, then what he calls State or 'professorial' philosophy, and now science have been used as justifications for some people to exploit others. With the clarity and percipience which are so characteristic of his writing, and with a relevance which has if anything increased in the hundred years since he wrote it, he suggests, for example, that the much-vaunted impartiality of science is merely a smokescreen for the operation of interest:

> Contemporary science investigates facts.
>
> But what facts? Why those particular facts and not others?
>
> Scientists of today are very fond of saying solemnly and confidently: 'We only investigate facts,' imagining these words to have some meaning. One cannot possibly only investigate facts for the number of facts available for investigation is *innumerable* (in the exact sense of that word). Before investigating the facts one must have a theory on the basis of which such or such facts are selected from among the innumerable quantity.

And, of course, as Tolstoy goes on to point out, the theory is one which happens to justify the social *status quo*. A few pages further on, he also indicates the selective nature of our intellectual interests.

*L. Tolstoy, *What Then Must We Do?* First published 1886.

17

Citing the influence of Comte's philosophical positivism on the new enthusiasm for science, he writes:

> What is remarkable . . . is that of Comte's works, which consist of two parts – the positive philosophy and the positive politics – the learned world only accepted the first: the part which on the new experimental basis, offered a justification for the existing evil of human societies; but the second part, dealing with the moral obligations of altruism resulting from acknowledging humanity as an organism, was considered not merely unimportant but even insignificant and unscientific.

I do not believe that anyone who attends closely to the nature of ordinary people's distress – even if it appears to be 'purely psychological' – and confronts honestly the resistance of its causes to our efforts at magical cure, can ultimately ignore the fundamental part played in our suffering by the disavowed (repressed) operation of interest on a societal scale. Explanations of distress which rely simply on concepts of the malfunctioning or intransigence of individuals in fact lead nowhere, unless, that is, explainers and explained manage to collude in an illusory version of a world which has no substance outside our own heads. We have developed and exhausted just about every variation on the theme of either individual mechanical breakdown or personal moral inadequacy to account for the anxiety, isolation, fear, depression and frustration which are endemic in our society, so far with no convincing success. There is, for example, no satisfactory evidence that 'mental illnesses' are illnesses at all, but there is every indication that our pain, confusion, suspicion and hostility, the vulnerability which we try to disguise in so many desperate and crazy ways, arise out of our conduct towards each other.

No matter how appalling the circumstances in which people live, it seems that sooner or later they grow accustomed to them. Not only that, but it seems quite quickly that these are the only possible circumstances which *could* exist. When one thinks of the contrasts which are to be found in the world between the ways of life of the people in it, it is in many ways astonishing that people so readily accept their lot. For example, both the most and the least privileged are quite likely to view their circumstances as *both* inevitable *and* somehow deserved. In this manner, when people seek an explanation for their unhappy situation, they tend to seek it in some kind of *natural* rather than *social* order. This propensity of human beings, whatever its fundamental explanation, is one which it is very easy to exploit, often unconsciously, in the interests of those so disposed, and one of the best ways of exploiting it is by creating institutions (like 'scientific psychology') which reinforce our readiness to believe that our unhappiness is the natural result of our personal shortcomings.

It is strangely difficult for the naive investigator (and no investigators are to be found more naive than those in psychology and psychiatry) to uncover the principles by which modern Western society seems to render so many of its members so desperately unhappy. One reason for this difficulty is that the naive investigator is as prone as anyone else to take society as given and to focus on the problem of how individuals may be brought to 'adjust' to it. However, naivety may to some extent be overcome by an (all too rare) combination of experience and honesty, in which case it becomes clear that the individuals cannot be taken out of the context of the society which they inhabit.

Slowly one becomes led to see that the hostile defensiveness which so often characterizes our relations with each other, the heartless ways in which we exploit and use each other, the extent to which we accept and reject ourselves and each other as commodities, *entirely inescapably* reflect the culture in which we live. One can no more easily opt out of a culture than one can opt out of a physical environment, and a poisonous culture will affect one just as surely as will a polluted atmosphere.

Encapsulated in our belief that the reasons for our conduct are to be tracked down somewhere inside our own skulls, most of us assume that, if life becomes uncomfortable, it must be some individual's 'fault'. Most psychotherapy patients, for example, are quite surprised, if greatly relieved, to discover that their predicament is not unique in the therapist's experience. What, to the attentive therapist, comes as even more surprising is the discovery that not only are patients' experiences and 'problems' often not unique, *they are general*, and more than likely pretty familiar in the therapist's personal experience as well. As I shall discuss in greater detail in Chapter 6, this is nowhere clearer than in our 'relationship problems'. What seems to millions of men and women a singularly personal and isolating misery, a purely private mixture of hate, rejection and despair, is in fact being experienced (or repressed) in one form or another in practically every household in the land. We are caught up in the movements of our culture as droplets in a wave. This is not to say that we have no unique difficulties or purely individual 'problems', but that very much more often than it seems our predicament is created by circumstances we all share but none of us is able to see or to acknowledge. Recognition of this state of affairs has the most profound implications, since it opens the way for hatred, bitterness, recrimination, guilt and self-disgust to be replaced by, at least, a kind of sympathetic tolerance for those who are, in Dickens's phrase, our 'fellow passengers to the grave'.

Culture does not come about by accident. Just as the psychotherapist may after long and patient inquiry, perhaps with the aid of one or two fortuitous discoveries, slowly begin to be able to formulate an idea of the patient's unacknowledged reasons for his or her conduct, so may one at the wider, societal level begin to see – almost by becoming aware of the factors we explicitly *do not* refer to – what some of the reasons may be for our adherence to our 'psycho-noxious' ways of life. Most of these reasons, it seems to me, cluster around a collective aim to maximize, at more or less any cost (to others), personal interest. We are united nowhere more than in our selfishness.

When our fundamental collective aim is less than worthy, we construct special institutions for the more or less sole (if quite unconscious) purpose of repressing its recognition. Psychiatry and psychology largely fulfil this role, and so it is not surprising that the discussion of interest forms virtually no part of their concern. One has, rather, to turn to social criticism within history for the beginnings of an understanding of what our inarticulate projects may be.

It is almost certainly as misleading to look back on former times as less problematic or destructive than ours as it is to regard our own times as the inevitable achievement of progress. However, there seems to be a strong case to be made for the reflection that for the past four to five hundred years Western society has become less and less concerned with a social order based on moral principles and more and more concerned with one based on economic principles. It would of course be utterly false to regard the Middle Ages as a period when no one had an interest in power and riches, but there seems to be at least a measure of agreement among historians that some coherence was then lent to society by an explicit, largely religious philosophy which aimed at the moral regulation of people's conduct towards each other, and which indeed had some success in defining a social order in which everyone had rights as well as obligations. Though exploitation and corruption may have been rife, it is still worth noting that, as R. H. Tawney pithily puts it:

If it is proper to insist on the prevalence of avarice and greed in high places, it is not less important to observe that men called these vices by their right names, and had not learned to persuade themselves that greed was enterprise and avarice economy.*

It seems a long way from the experience of distress of individual people in psychotherapy to reflections concerning the undermining of ecclesiastical authority at the time of the Renaissance and the subsequent rise to power of a class of merchants and financiers who were to change the sin of usury into the virtue of profit. And yet I believe that the connection is inescapable, and I find myself unexpectedly grateful to historians who, like Tawney, throw light on the societal conditions in which our experience is set, and which go some considerable way towards exposing the reasons for its so-frequently distressing nature. For while it would be at best tendentious and at worst entirely misleading to attempt to derive a psychology of individual experience from an account of historical processes, it seems much more intellectually reassuring to find in the historical account explanations for individual experience which would remain otherwise quite unexplainable.

Most psychologists work within a ludicrously short time scale. The 'literature' of research and 'laboratory experiment' by means of which most British and American psychologists orientate themselves tends to be compressed within – to put it on the generous side – the most recent twenty years. Satisfaction with this state of affairs depends upon a confidence in the relative infallibility of the 'scientific' methodology of 'objective' measurement and 'quantification' of human 'behaviour', and an indifference to the influence of historical, social and political factors, which seem to me to be becoming increasingly hard to maintain. The necessary alternative is, then, to stray outside the bounds of one's own discipline, and gladly to accept from whatever other sources offer themselves the kinds of conceptual help which contribute to making sense of one's experience. At a time when intellectual specialization is so narrow that 'education' in one branch of 'knowledge' qualifies one not at all to judge the validity of argument in other branches, such straying beyond one's 'legitimate' boundaries is not without risk. However, since this kind of specialization is one of the consequences of the workings of interest in the very way that I am seeking to criticize, it is a risk I shall from time to time have to take.

In trying to understand the frequently quite unconscious aims of individuals it often helps to ignore what they say, to themselves as well as to us, and to look as ingenuously as possible at what

*R. H. Tawney, *Religion and the Rise of Capitalism*, Penguin Books, 1938.

they seem to be trying to do, in which case the aims may become quite surprisingly obvious. In the same way, if one wants fully to comprehend the impetus behind our collective, social conduct, one need often do no more than ignore the rhetoric and look instead at our actions. Such ingenuous observation only goes to confirm the ubiquity of interest. We have carried the commercial values developed over the last five centuries, at first with shame and later with enthusiasm, to a point where all our dealings with each other, at the institutional as much as if not more than at the personal level, are based on the advantages which are likely to accrue in terms of power and money. Socially, politically, recreationally, intellectually, educationally and academically, in every sphere and department of life, it is towards money and its power that our conduct is orientated.

There is still a *touch* of shame about this. Though our fascination with the struggle for money-power is only too evident to the most casual observer, we still often tend to hide it behind a moralistic screen of judgments of good and bad, and in this are not unlike our Puritan ancestor described by Tawney:

> Convinced that character is all and circumstances nothing, he sees in the poverty of those who fall by the way, not a misfortune to be pitied and relieved, but a moral failing to be condemned, and in riches, not an object of suspicion — though like other gifts they may be abused — but the blessing which rewards the triumph of energy and will. Tempered by self-examination, self-discipline, self-control, he is the practical ascetic, whose victories are won not in the cloister, but on the battlefield, in the counting-house, and in the market.

In recent years, our love of money and confidence in the values of the market place, the primacy of cost-benefit analysis to moral questions of right and wrong, have become more overt, as has our readiness to expend each other, sacrifice our young and discard our old in our personal interest. But even still there is a tendency to disavow our intentions, or at least to draw a veil of repression over our most basic inclinations.

The crude, 'value-free', 'objective' and mechanistic preoccupations of 'modern science' have of course done much both to obscure the nature of our enterprise and to lend it an authority which might otherwise be less easy to establish. This is certainly the case with psychology, which serves with studied innocence to divert our gaze from our least creditable undertakings. An examination of the indexes of the nine textbooks of psychology to be found in our local university book shop reveals that only three mention 'power' and *none* mention 'money'. How seriously should one take a 'science' which claims to deal with 'motivation' and the 'prediction and control of human behaviour' and yet which fails to mention the one most powerful motivator in every Western person's life? (The answer should probably be *very* seriously, since psychology is clearly about something quite other than a *disinterested* examination of 'what makes us tick', and it is presumably important to know what that something other may be.)

It is my belief, then, that to trace the sources of what we feel as our individual distress, we shall need to turn to a critical examination of what our collective enterprises are. The intertwining of our interest with our dreams is leading us into a progressive carelessness of each other's welfare, to an extent indeed which will, *at the very best*, damage us for generations to come.

2

The Pursuit of Happiness

It seems a matter of self-evidence to most people (indeed I wonder if, in our hearts, *any* of us can escape such a view) that the point of life is to be happy. If, in an attempt to tap a relatively selfless opinion, you ask people what they would most want for the lives of their actual or hypothetical children, they will usually say 'happiness'. They may also specify other conditions, like health, material success or a modest degree of fame, upon which happiness may be taken to depend. Not everybody chooses happiness, but most people do, and in the highly informal 'experiments' I have made in asking people this question there seem to be no unusual patterns to the responses they give in terms of age, sex, class, etc.

And yet, in some ways, to hold happiness as the ideal of life seems to me to involve a number of difficulties and paradoxes, not the least of which is the extreme infrequency with which, despite all our best efforts, it seems to be achieved. We appear to be surprisingly undaunted by disappointment. Infrequency of achievement does not in itself, of course, render the ideal of happiness invalid in any way, but it does among other things add an element almost of cruelty to the pursuit of our elusive goal.

Further reflection leads one to wonder whether the attainment of happiness may be so infrequent because in fact it is not even possible. How, for example, does one know that one has reached the point in one's life where happiness has been achieved? What does one do with it when one has got it? Can one specify the conditions in which it may be retained? Can one see what other people need to do to gain it, perhaps being able to draw up a kind of blueprint for the achievement of general happiness?

Even if one cannot easily arrive at a formula for the capture of happiness in the present, it may be misleadingly simple to imagine what a human life in which ultimate happiness has been reached might look like, and those of us who have found the early and middle years of life less rewarding in terms of happiness than perhaps we had hoped as children, can still probably fantasize how we may yet grasp it in our declining years. The 'happiness' which throughout our lives stayed just beyond our reach becomes, in the nick of time, the 'fulfilment' of old age. Our faded gaze rests with contentment on the persons of those who love us and who accept from us with gratitude the fruits of a mellowed wisdom as they enact in our autumnal world the little dramas we ourselves have known so well. I have read about such old people, but I have never met one, and unless it is possible that a lifetime's isolation in some privileged enclave could somehow preserve a person from knowledge of the world outside, any such 'fulfilled' departure from this earth would seem to me to involve, at the very least, an extraordinarily egocentric self-satisfaction. Perhaps a merciful old age would temper our 'rage at the dying of the light', but I hope would not obliterate it, or transform it into a kind of fatuous contentment simply because there is no further chance of influencing events.

And so, a further paradox: if we got 'happiness', would we want it? To take for a moment the extreme case, it is hard to conceive of any version of everlasting, perhaps heavenly existence (in this world or the next) which would not become intolerably burdensome; there could be no more boring place than paradise. The enormously powerful attraction of 'happiness' lies in the fact that (in the commodified form in which we conceive of it) we *never* experience it, it is *always* just beyond our grasp. Happiness, of the kind which can be pursued, is an illusion.

One may ask people a slightly more awkward question than that concerning what they would want in life for their children. Imagine that you are visited shortly before the birth of your only child by an archangel who offers you a choice you cannot decline: either your child will grow to a great age, loved and respected by all, having done no wrong or mean thing to anybody, successful, rich, healthy, and, above all, happy, *but* will have made no memorable contribution to the future of the species beyond the immediate good works of a lifetime. *Or,* your child will have a short, bitter life, full of spiritual pain and bodily ill-health, will be universally misunderstood and rejected, *but* will make through his or her work a contribution which will prove to be of fundamental, beneficial significance to the culture for centuries to come. Which would you choose?

My own experience is that people have little hesitation over choosing one or the other of these hypothetical futures for their hypothetical offspring, and that the vast majority plump for the happiness option. To get a reasonably honest answer, the question has, obviously, to be posed innocently, but even those people who angrily sense some moral disapprobation of their choice of happiness, still, very understandably, defend it on the grounds that *whatever* their hypothetical child's potential achievement, they could not wish upon him or her the kind of unhappiness the archangel promises.

Hypothetical games such as these are of course predictive of nothing and revealing of very little, and though one can add a surface plausibility to this example by, for instance, citing the life of Mozart, there is in fact no *necessary* connection between ill-health, rejection, etc., and creativity. Indeed, it is a central contention of this book that constructively creative and socially valuable conduct is most likely to be fostered by the kind of concern for their children's well-being which loving parents characteristically show. In other words, the archangel's offer forces a *false* choice, and it is probably that which causes a measure of irritation in some of those who respond to it. Nevertheless, what *is* revealed, I think, by the large preponderance of happiness choices people seem to make, is the extent to which we implicitly believe in the values of an illusion. This is, of course, no surprising discovery, but merely confirms what is already entirely obvious to the most casual observer of our ways of life. What seems to motivate us, to keep us going from day to day, is the pursuit of happiness; and yet, if 'pursuable happiness' is necessarily an illusion which can only melt in one's grasp as soon as one's fingers close around it, how can its enormous force as a motivator for human conduct be accounted for? Why is it so hard for people to be able even to imagine any other point to life than the personal satisfaction of the individuals living it?

Among the many factors which might contribute to an answer to these questions, there are two to which I want to give prominence. The first refers to an inevitable feature of every person's embodied experience – the memory of bliss. The second refers to a practically inescapable feature of our society, and one without which it would rapidly crumble and be transformed – the profitability of illusion.

It is a fact not lost on students of individual psychology – most notably Freud – that our first and most blissful experience of happiness is probably also our last. It is a virtually universal tragedy of human experience that the very earliest impressions we have should be those of such perfect warmth and protectedness and oneness (with the mother), both inside and for a while probably outside the womb, that we may be tempted to spend the rest of our lives trying to recreate what is in fact an unrepeatable situation. By the time we have become reasonably competent in the use of language, that experience of perfect happiness has probably been overlaid by much harsher realities, and since what we normally consider as memory depends upon our ability to rehearse experiences in words, our 'memory' of bliss is not something we can get to grips with in our thoughts, but remains in our bodies as a kind of aching absence. Those of our experiences which are beyond the reach of words, when their bodily 'memory' is stirred by some perhaps fortuitous set of circumstances, tend to be rekindled in a kind of awe-filled burst of inexpressible, unnameably familiar ecstasy. (Such an experience is falling in love, but, in some ways sadly, as we must grow out of infancy, so we must grow out of being-in-love.)

Those psychologists who tend towards a view of human development as a kind of mechanical unfolding of an inevitable series of stages of experience are likely to see the tragic frustration of the infant's initial experience of bliss as a *particularly* inescapable and particularly constant feature of our psychology, and in this they are unlikely to be wrong. But even so we would do well to remember that the individual's experience is set within a social context, and the extent of his or her disillusionment, and certainly the degree of its painfulness, will depend quite largely on the provision which is made for it.* Does one, for example, speed the process of severance from maternal love in the belief that the sooner the child learns to cope with a hard, tough life the better, or does one gently protect its tenderness and vulnerability until it has matured to a point where one feels that it can take on for itself the unkindnesses of the world? No doubt both answers, as well as complete indifference to the question, have been popular at various junctures in our recent as well as our more distant history. For the moment, however, what I want to highlight are the *uses* to which we have put our 'memory' of bliss. It seems to me, indeed, that assiduity in *making use of* the aching absence of fundamental happiness has been far greater than any attempt rationally to understand the painful passions associated with it and to construct a social world which treats them with sympathetic kindness; the brave efforts of some psychologists in this latter direction have, after all, met with little respect.

The very unrepeatability of that first experience of radical protectedness and passivity, the effortless achievement (for a while) of unlimited warmth, gratification and love, has been exploited in our culture to fuel an endlessly tantalizing hope. We know, in some sense, that that state is attainable (for once we really did experience it) and so we easily fall prey to the promise of its reoccurrence. It is precisely the 'pursuit of happiness' – culturally sanctioned at the very highest levels – which holds out this promise to us. But the actuality of its nature as an illusion, the fact that our infantile experience is unrepeatable, ensures that we do not attain it, and so we are left in unending and empty pursuit. All the time we see as just beyond our grasp what is in fact not there at all. And the more that 'happiness' and 'success' elude us, the harder we strive to overtake them.

There is a bleak view to be taken of this state of affairs, which,

---

*In this connection see I. D. Suttie, *The Origins of Love and Hate*, Penguin Books, 1960.

as with Freud's 'death instinct', suggests that our futile pursuit of effortless gratification leads us eventually to seek the everlasting, if negative peace of death. Nor is this view to be dismissed lightly, for there is much that argues in its favour. We do indeed seem to pursue our fantasies of inert, passive satisfaction beyond the boundaries of fiction and dream. 'Scientists' actually have experimented with the idea of stimulation of 'pleasure centres' within the brain as an attractive way of passing our time,* and there are people who do not regard as preposterous or even disturbing the idea of a *totally* self-sufficient person living a life of sensual bliss alone in a glass bubble. One only has to look at the world-wide success of the American junk food industry,

> That is, the drink-down, quick-sugar foods of spoiled children, and the pre-cut meat for lazy chewing beloved of ages six to ten. Nothing is bitten or bitten-off, very little is chewed; there is a lot of sugar for animal energy, but not much solid food to grow on†

to see the attractions of a return to infancy, and by extension to the womb. And it is by no means implausible to project one further step to complete oblivion as part of our unconscious craving.

And yet – I hope, at least – this is not a *necessary* feature of our individual psychology, but an only *potentially* fatal weakness brought about by our early experience of bliss. For if this is a weakness to which the very structure of our bodies exposes us, it is still one which occurs in a world which may or may not encourage it. Though weaknesses are indeed likely to be exploited, they may also be acknowledged, understood, and even, eventually, turned into strengths.

It does indeed seem that we pursue an illusory happiness with all the futile enthusiasm of a tame mouse in a treadmill – but how is it that we could be so blind? Rather than simply being misled by some intrinsic weakness of psychological structure, we are, I believe, blinded by interest. There is money to be made from the pursuit of happiness.

I do not wish to suggest that there is anything *fundamentally* wrong with the idea of happiness: it is clearly preferable for people to be happy rather than unhappy, and there is no *necessary* connection between virtue and misery. There have been times in our history when the pursuit of happiness seemed an altogether less hollow undertaking than it does today. For example, it is not

---

*For a particularly disturbing account of one such experiment, see Chapter 2 of my *Psychotherapy: A Personal Approach*, Dent, 1978.
†Goodman, op. cit.

difficult to detect in the writers of the Enlightenment and in the philosophical and political works of the British Utilitarians (i.e. those late eighteenth- and early nineteenth-century thinkers who believed that 'good' could be measured in terms of 'happiness') a spirit of real hopefulness and generosity as they glimpsed the possibility of constructing an unprecedentedly equitable society in which happiness – freedom from want as well as political representation and influence – might be spread as widely as possible.

It seems, however, always to be the case that significant movements in our cultural and political history, particularly those which open up liberating vistas of change, even 'progress', last but a brief instant before their motivating ideas and the institutions they create are put to the use of those who have the power to turn them to their interest. One can think of several examples. Christ's revolutionary teaching concerning personal responsibility and love, and the example of his life, were almost immediately turned into an oppressive church orthodoxy which established a doctrine of myth and magic and a coercive political power which were to betray truly Christian values for centuries. Relative freedom from the sclerotic and corrupt power of a decadent Church offered Renaissance man a glimpse of what it would be like to organize life on the basis of scientific reason and subjective authority, but it was not to be long before science – at least in terms of its intellectually liberating vision – became a travesty of itself, and man's momentary apprehension of self-responsibility was quickly usurped by the State in combination with a 'reformed' religious hypocrisy, and turned against him. Much the same seems to have been the case with the Enlightened vision of happiness.

It seems as though the new-found freedom of a prosperous middle class for a while imbued it with a generous impulse to share its good fortune with those who were, as in contrast with the landed aristocracy it had itself also so recently been, less privileged. John Passmore puts it well:*

> The Enlighteners . . . thought they knew who was bound to come to overt power in the State – the commercial classes. And there was, they were convinced, a natural alliance between the new governors and the spirit of enlightenment. Overt power to the middle class, actual power to the intellectuals – that was the future of society as they envisaged it. The 'honest man', the merchant, the 'civically good' man, replaced the aristocrat and the hero – in England especially – as the 'ideal type' of humanity.

*J. Passmore, *The Perfectibility of Man*, Duckworth, 1970.

And:

> Commerce and liberty, so Voltaire maintained in his *Philosophical Letters*, are intimately associated. The close link between literature and finance was, he thought, one of the glories of the eighteenth century. No Rotarian could be more enthusiastic about the benefits of commerce than was Joseph Priestley. By bringing the merchant into contact with other places and people, he tells us, commerce 'tends greatly to expand the mind and to cure us of many hurtful prejudices'; it encourages benevolence and a love of peace; it develops such virtues as punctuality and 'the principals of strict justice and honour' . . . 'Men of wealth and influence', so he sums up, 'who act upon the principles of virtue and religion, and conscientiously make their power subservient to the good of their country, are the men who are the greatest honour to human nature, and the greatest blessing to human societies.'

A connection between big business and philanthropy would be unlikely to be one impressing itself upon modern intellectual observers of society, although of course it is one which big business seeks, through procedures of 'image building', to create. Once again, those processes which at the time looked to constitute a liberating move and were advocated with enthusiastic optimism by those caught up in it, came very rapidly to be exploited in the sole interests of those – now the 'bourgeoisie' – with power.

It is instructive in this respect to reflect upon the career of the most 'official' sanction we have to pursue happiness. It was of course Thomas Jefferson who first articulated 'the pursuit of happiness' as one of the rights of men in the American Declaration of Independence. According to Hannah Arendt,* however, Jefferson himself may at that time not have been entirely clear about what he meant by the phrase, and his idea of happiness and ours may well have diverged considerably in the intervening two hundred years. She argues that by 'happiness' he may have meant, at least partly, what he meant elsewhere when he wrote of 'public happiness', that is the freedom of people to take part in their political self-determination. However, as she points out, the phrase

> was almost immediately deprived of its double sense and understood as the right of citizens to pursue their personal interests and thus to act according to the rules of private self-interest. And these rules, whether they spring from dark

*H. Arendt, *On Revolution*, Penguin Books, 1973.

desires of the heart or from the obscure necessities of the household, have never been notably 'enlightened'.

Arendt suggests also that in debates in the Assembly

> none of the delegates would have suspected the astonishing career of this 'pursuit of happiness', which was to contribute more than anything else to a specifically American ideology, to the terrible misunderstanding that, in the words of Howard Mumford Jones, holds that men are entitled to 'the ghastly privilege of pursuing a phantom and embracing a delusion'.

Arising out of this discussion, then, are two possible views, or versions of happiness: happiness as something which may attend or follow from our actions (as for example in the conduct of our political freedom, our ability to take part in the affairs of our own government), and happiness as something 'in itself' which may be pursued. In fact, Arendt suggests that the (illusory) pursuit of happiness as a thing in itself, and of the associated ideals of 'abundance and endless consumption', are the product of a vision conditioned by poverty, and it is for that reason that they are so characteristic of American culture, since it was that country which seemed to promise so much to the poor emigrants from Europe:

> The hidden wish of poor men is not 'To each according to his needs', but 'to each according to his desires'. And while it is true that freedom can only come to those whose needs have been fulfilled, it is equally true that it will escape those who are bent upon living for their desires. The American dream, as the nineteenth and twentieth centuries under the impact of mass immigration came to understand it, was . . . unhappily, the dream of a 'promised land' where milk and honey flow. And the fact that the development of modern technology was so soon able to realize this dream beyond anyone's wildest expectation quite naturally had the effect of confirming for the dreamers that they really had come to live in the best of all possible worlds.

Now that America has successfully sold its dream to most of the rest of the world, those of us in Europe who have become, as it were, the all-too-willing subjects of an economic and cultural empire based on the values of which Arendt is rightly so contemptuous, can no longer stand by (as we seemed only a few years ago to be able to do) with amusement or disbelief as we watch the tasteless antics of our trans-Atlantic relatives. For we are now busily performing the self-same antics. We have bought, lock, stock and barrel, the idea of happiness as commodity, and we pursue it with singleminded dedication.

The increasing affluence and freedom from want of 'developed' Western society has, however, not resulted in our seeing through the illusory nature of our pursuit of happiness, and the reason for this lies presumably in the changed nature of our enslavement. The interests of power no longer lie, as until recently they so transparently did, in extracting from an oppressed work force the maximum production at the minimum cost, but in stimulating from a dazed and pacified population the maximum consumption at the greatest price the market will bear. The chief means by which this may be achieved are through the promotion of happiness as a commodity and the prevention of happiness as a consequence, or epiphenomenon, of activity.

Anyone who has tried to do it – and that must, surely, include everyone – knows how impossible it is to manufacture happiness. Whether or not one is happy depends entirely upon events and circumstances which one cannot will, and usually the more self-consciously one attempts to be happy, the more signally one fails. When happiness does arise, it does so spontaneously and unbidden, and often unexpectedly, as a concomitant, usually, of our absorbed and unself-conscious activity. It arises out of doing things, or out of our doing things together, and it is often only after we have ceased doing them that we realize we were happy. Those who recognize this are easily led to romanticize the lives of people who are necessarily committed to endless hard work, punctuated only occasionally by simple festivals or the innocent pleasures of family celebrations, but such is not my intention. I rather doubt if the peasant's long-awaited appointment with a happy Christmas is any more often successful than the culmination of our own harassed and jaded preparations for that same event. Unremitting drudgery is likely to be no more rewarding than the apathetic killing of time and invention of 'pleasurable' sensations necessitated by satiated affluence. Happiness comes, rather, from having something useful and absorbing and demanding to do which can be valued by the doer as well as those for whom he or she is doing it.

It is this form of happiness which has become vanishingly rare in our world, and in my view it is the lack of the possibility for this form of happiness which, at least as much as anything else, lies behind our despair. We have constructed a society which is in essence a vast machine designed for the maintenance and development of an illusion. We believe that the value of our lives may be measured by the degree of their happiness and that happiness in its turn may be understood as personal satisfaction and fulfilment, to be gained, if not *through* the acquisition of things, then certainly *as* the acquisition of things. In these beliefs we are misled on the one hand by the technological pragmatism we have developed over the past four centuries and on the other by our enthusiasm for greedy exploitation. Our technological bent has led us to isolate the happiness we have rightly observed as occasionally accompanying our activity, to posit it as the point of life, and then to try to manufacture it as a commodity. Our greed has led us, freed from the repressive moral strictures of a 'parental' religious authority, to throw ourselves upon the world's bounty with all the lack of restraint of a group of adolescents at their first party. And, of course, our genius for exploitation has quickly revealed that our unrestrained adolescent greed offers a market for ever more 'exciting' and 'satisfying' commodities which may be tended and stoked and stimulated more or less endlessly. Rather than being, as it were, encouraged by our social and cultural institutions to grow out of our infantile craving for the delights of the womb and the breast towards a mature and sober undertaking of a contribution to the life of our society and the continuation of our species, it has become our aim to benefit in every way possible from a concerted pandering to our longing for blissful satiation. We all believe in happiness, and most of us have a stake in its production and consumption. We thus become caught up in a frenzied pursuit of happiness which, being illusory, renders us ever more dazed and out of touch with our embodied reality, and ever more vulnerable to and injured by the abuses of our exploitation of each other.

People suffer bitterly, go crazy and even kill themselves because (among other reasons) they are unhappy. It is easy to see why: to be unhappy means in our society to have lost the point of living. (In making this point I do not wish to justify unhappiness nor to advocate the policy of the stiff upper lip. All too often unhappiness is seen as something some people have to get used to so that other people can escape it. This constitutes a version of moralism about which I shall say more in the final chapter.) The *inevitable* non-achievement of the greedy individualistic satiation which we take to signify happiness, means that we suffer from a kind of collective, chronic frustration.

In the very midst of a kind of lunatic celebration of symbolic satisfactions, a mirage of pleasures excited and achieved, people are in fact almost beside themselves with need. A sense of despairing neediness seems to me to be endemic at all levels of our society – experienced just as much by the 'helpers' as by those they seek to help – and to lie curled at the centre of most 'relationships'. For our frantic search for happiness meets only emptiness, and if we could we would all scream like abandoned infants as our mouths fail to encounter the promised breast. We are, however, not infants, but rather adolescents who don't know our own strength, and the response to our frustration is more likely to be a destructive lashing-out than an infantile scream.

Happiness – of any kind, commodity or 'epiphenomenon' – cannot be the point of life. Indeed, the very expectation that there must be a discernible point to life constitutes the first step towards a life-denying individualism in which the future of the species becomes sacrificed to personal immortality.* Among the reasons for our reluctance to abandon our pursuit of happiness, however, is the fact that so many of us make a living by encouraging it. But abandon it we must if we are to progress beyond a struggle with illusory unhappiness, grief at the lack of blissful satisfaction, to a struggle with the causes of real unhappiness – the injuries we do each other as we exploit and compete with each other for what we take to be the good things of life.

Whatever their circumstances in life, it is, as I have already noted, hard for most people to imagine that they could be otherwise. Even people living in squalor and misery do not necessarily *know* that they are, and anyone proclaiming a vision of a better life may have considerable difficulty persuading unhappy people that they are indeed unhappy. This is not as paradoxical as it seems, as any psychotherapist, for example, should know: the 'neurotic' patient's suffering is most often inarticulate and its causes unacknowledged; he or she has to be *brought to see* what the trouble – with the world and with his or her relation to it – really is. A condition of political repression has always been that it is able to thrive on the unawareness of the people it oppresses that they are indeed oppressed, and those of broader vision who are able to envisage a life of liberty may have to struggle hard to get their view accepted.

To suggest, therefore, that our current ways of life distort almost beyond recognition what human existence should look like, and that our relations with each other and the world constrict and mutilate our experience, our potentialities and our actual living presence, is likely to be met by blank incredulity and scorn. To protect us against any such view (apart from the usual processes of resistance to change which will be discussed in Chapter 5) we have on the one hand the whole apparatus of marketing of an illusory happiness and on the other such a familiarity with the

---

*It is significant in this respect that even so humane and critically gifted a believer in the greatest happiness for the greatest number as William Godwin (see his *Enquiry Concerning Political Justice*, 1793) should have fallen for a Utopian fantasy of man as non-reproductive and immortal. There are no doubt millions today who would see nothing the matter with that as an ideal for the future.

conditions of our crippled lives that we take them for an ineluctable normality.

Nevertheless, almost anyone, if he or she can bear to look, will catch a glimpse from time to time of the ways in which we have sold ourselves into slavery, of the sad results of having done so, and indeed of the devices whereby we prevent ourselves from seeing what we have done.

Just at the most obvious level, a weakening of our individualistic and tribal values would allow us to see how our personal, commodified happiness is bought, and always has been bought, at the expense of others. The evidence of the results of our having unloaded our want and discomfort on to others — other classes, races, nations, even continents — is absolutely plain for us to see, if only in our own inner cities. Sometimes, certainly (as in the case at the present time with starvation in Africa) our compassion is stirred, but even then only rarely do we see that 'their' problems cannot be disentangled from our conduct. Hannah Arendt points out* how even the civilized prosperity of revolutionary America was built upon the grotesque values of slavery. Again, it is common to represent the 'problems' of Western 'civilization' as those which naturally follow upon affluence: we have conquered want, and must now concentrate upon our spiritual and therapeutic needs and cultivate the values of 'fun' and leisure. This kind of view, probably wearing a little thin now after its particular popularity in the sixties, is plausible only if we manage to disregard, i.e. repress, at least half the consequences of our actions: we have not conquered want, but merely discovered ways of exporting it.

The peculiar dishonesty of repression also haunts our more personal experience, numbing the pain we would otherwise feel at the destruction of human potential we witness in our lives more or less as a matter of course. How easily, for example, the middle-aged person comes to accept with only a minimum of sorrow the almost standard transformation of the children he or she once knew: open, inquisitive four and five-year-olds, bearing the clearly visible buds of whole ranges of ability and concern, become now uniform, already half-hopeless nineteen- and twenty-year-olds, cynical devotees of commodified sex and bad music, defensive about their feelings and encapsulated in a world bounded by consumption. I know there are exceptions, but too few, surely, to justify anything other (if only we could but feel it) than a sickened rage at the sort of society we have created.

One has often to make a special effort of the imagination to see quite how mad and destructive the world we live in has become.

*On Revolution, op. cit.

This is only a seeming paradox, indicating more a deep and usually unquestioning familiarity with our environment than any reassuring possibility that things are not really all that bad. The effort of imagination needed is like that which dreamers make in order to wake themselves from a nightmare.

Insights sometimes present themselves at the most unexpected times and places. For example, a young waiter in one of those mass-produced Italian restaurants paces across the fake ceramic floor, gliding from narrow hips, swaying broad shoulders. He tosses his thick black hair so that it quivers on the collar of his open shirt, and glances semi-boldly and semi-defensively at the two girls who are waiting for their food at a corner table. He has perhaps ten paces to walk from the centre of the restaurant to the bar where the pizzas are being made. Every step of the way he is utterly conscious of himself, of his luxuriant mane, his olive skin, his narrow hips. He is a tall, strong young man caged in a pretend environment, serving day in and day out the same junk food to an endless stream of customers for whom the most he may hope to be is the object of an idle admiration or desire.

In those rare moments when the familiar world (for example of waiters and restaurants) breaks open to reveal how much worse things are than they appear, the accompanying emotion seems usually to be one of sadness. The waiter is not obviously hurt by his world, and one feels neither sorrow nor contempt for him, nor even anger at the circumstances which have conspired to make a mockery of a life which would, one feels (no doubt sentimentally), have been more suitably spent less self-consciously among vines or olive groves. For a moment, rather, he becomes a symbol of us all, and his (and our) unawareness of his (and our) plight, our acceptance of what we all too easily see as 'reality', is above all *sad*.

I remember, years ago, watching the chimps at London Zoo. A small crowd had gathered to watch them disport themselves in their 'outdoor' cage. Two of them swung into a smoothly practised routine: in an almost single movement of flowing synchrony one ran along the upper branch of a dead tree which lay in the cage while the other entwined itself gracefully round a horizontal branch perhaps six feet lower. The reclining chimp arched back his head, and at that precise moment the chimp on the upper branch, with pin-point accuracy, urinated into his open mouth. The crowd gasped with surprise and laughed with a mixture of disgust and admiration at the virtuosity of the performance, and the chimps looked towards their audience with unmistakable delight and pride.

I suspect that a lot of what passes for 'human nature' is really the result of our having to deal with a certain *kind* of world. Self-consciousness, for example, whether in the form of vanity or shyness (both of which are *characteristic* of our time), might not seem so inevitable in a world which gave us space in which to *do* things.

If the possibility is denied you of doing anything of value in the world, you have to use your ingenuity in order to feel alive while passing the time. If your activity counts for nothing your *person* is likely to become salient – it will become important what you look like (you could decorate yourself, dye your hair) and what you feel like (you may become absorbed in the state of excitation or satiation of your nervous system, stimulation and satisfaction). In his savagely constricted and inexpressibly sad little environment at the zoo, Guy the gorilla passed much of his time in a rather distractedly off-hand indulgence in masturbation. Unlike the chimpanzees, he did not seem to mind what people thought, apparently not noticing their blushes and giggles.

It is really not the case that we treat animals differently from the way we treat each other: what is most disturbing about factory farming is its revelation of the mentality which lies behind it, and which is the same as that lying behind, for example, high-rise building. Point for point, the life of a battery hen is no different from that of the high-rise tenant. Both are victims of the same cruelty, indifference and greed, and in all probability neither is aware of it. Furthermore, the suffering occasioned by their enslavement will be met not with liberation, but with treatment.

Cruelty, indifference and greed are distributed throughout our society, and are not to be identified solely in the intentions or malicious motivation of any particular individuals or groups; I shall return to this question in future chapters.

I think I can remember a time (but perhaps I am deluding myself) when advertising was a distinctly suspect but sometimes faintly amusing undertaking in which fairly transparent lies were told about products which could not be relied upon to get sold on their own merits. Nowadays, however, we have developed a kind of commitment to the illusory nature of the artificial 'satisfactions' in which we imprison ourselves, and we seem therefore to stoke up a more and more frenetic and hyperbolic language by which to sell ourselves our self-deceiving vision. The advertising man becomes a symbol of the only kind of respectability which counts – the respectability of success – and his power to manufacture images is regarded, if not quite yet with awe, then certainly with uncritical admiration. The language of advertising and marketing infects just about every area of our activity as we persuade ourselves how 'important' and 'major' and 'exciting' our undertakings – academic and artistic as well as social and personal – are. The very language of international negotiation, in which 'front' men occupying jobs which might once have been filled by statesmen conduct 'propaganda battles' for the conquest of 'public opinion', becomes one of 'offers' in which 'fifty per cent reductions' (for example in nuclear weaponry) are bandied back and forth with all the gravity of cynical marketing executives whose function in life is to 'hype' poorly selling breakfast cereals. Even our most serious and vital concerns become in this way sucked into a kind of make-believe world in which 'credibility' counts more than life itself.

One's consciousness is relentlessly battered by the weaponry of image creation and fabricated excitement. Even a simple announcement of forthcoming programmes on the radio or television is uttered by a voice frenzied with fake enthusiasm, and our language is progressively emptied of subtlety and depth as every kind of activity possible or imaginable becomes reduced to its significance for how nice it will make us feel (you don't any longer so much 'have' or 'drink' a cup of coffee, for instance, as 'enjoy' it). It is impossible, particularly perhaps for a male, to walk through any city shopping or entertainment centre without coming under a kind of unremitting sexual assault: at every turn and corner another sexual image snatches at his flagging nervous system to associate with a flash of excitement some utterly sexually irrelevant object or service for sale. And the more habituated we become, the more lurid, basic or fantastic the sexual pitch is made. The everyday world we move in thus becomes one of ceaseless, frenetic, raucously euphoric promises of bliss. But we get used to it, and there are probably very few of us who do not take this crazy detachment from our actual embodied reality as normal.

> Commodity production and consumerism alter perceptions not just of the self but of the world outside the self. They create a world of mirrors, insubstantial images, illusions increasingly indistinguishable from reality. The mirror effect makes the subject an object; at the same time, it makes the world of objects an extension or projection of the self. It is misleading to characterize the culture of consumption as a culture dominated by things. The consumer lives surrounded not so much by things as by fantasies. He lives in a world that has no objective or independent existence and seems to exist only to gratify or thwart his desires.*

So that nothing may stand between us and the consumption of happiness, we are stripped of our functional activity and, like

*Christopher Lasch, *The Minimal Self. Psychic Survival in Troubled Times*, Picador, 1985.

battery animals, lifted from the course of time to be located in an endless present.

'A function may be defined as an activity which embodies and expresses the idea of social purpose.'* If life is not simply something for-oneself, to be enjoyed and indulged and spun out as long as possible (its dream-ideal thus being some form of solitary immortality), then its most profound value (and satisfaction) may come from the individual's being able, along with others, to make a contribution to – perform a function within – something infinitely larger than him- or herself. As part of an ever-evolving social process the individual is shaped by a largely unknown past and projected towards a totally unknowable future. Thus the individual becomes a tiny particle through which the course of social evolution moves; the meaning of our lives cannot be understood outside the context of the social and cultural processes in which they are embedded. It is probably misleading to speak of our bodies as having been designed *for* anything, but certainly if there is anything for which the design of our bodies is *suitable*, it is for contributing to a process far too great for us to be able to understand and a future far too distant and impenetrable for us to be able to divine. To see our bodies as being designed merely for the experience of pleasure or 'happiness' is surely to trivialize human existence to the point of utter despair.

> ... to say that the end of social institutions is happiness, is to say that they have no common end at all. For happiness is individual and to make happiness the object of society is to resolve society itself into the ambitions of numberless individuals, each directed towards the attainment of some personal purpose.
>
> Such societies may be called Acquisitive Societies, because their whole tendency and interest and preoccupation is to promote the acquisition of wealth. The appeal of this conception must be powerful, for it has laid the whole modern world under its spell.*

Human functions are, sadly, extremely vulnerable to exploitation by interest. Almost anything that people can do in the way of productive or creative work can be mechanized, objectified, appropriated and then sold back to them as passive consumers. The social activity of making music, for example, becomes the solitary reception of mass-produced sounds through headphones. Production becomes consumption, activity becomes spectacle. Even

*R. H. Tawney, *The Acquisitive Society*. First published 1921, Wheatsheaf Books, 1982.

relatively privileged functions of a service or professional nature (privileged in the sense that they are themselves not without an element of exploitation) may fall prey to the 'managerial' stratum of society which seeks to objectify and manipulate for profit just about any identifiable and potentially saleable form of human conduct. Anything people can do for themselves is the waste of an opportunity to make money, and it therefore becomes important to find ways of annexing the fruits of their activity and putting them up for sale. The medium through which the trick is performed is, of course, our fatal penchant for passivity, the blissful ease of inert consumption, but this would not have anything like the power over us it does were it not sanctioned by the values of a society (maintained through the more or less willing complicity of us all) which posits the making of money – 'the creation of wealth' – as the highest good, the necessity of necessities.

One can sell things only in the present. The past, from the salesman's point of view, is certainly a dead loss (hence the cultivation of obsolescence, the frenetic insistence on the 'now' and the 'new'), and the future is uncertain (hence the desperation to close the deal *today*). Happiness, therefore, becomes a phenomenon of the here and now. You must be satisfied, be excited, enjoy, have fun *now*. Every moment that passes in which your nervous system is not perceptibly going through the cycle of sensations involved in excitation/satisfaction is wasted, mis-spent (and unprofitable) time. Only new things matter; our pursuit of fulfilment *now* uproots us from our past and disconnects us from the things we knew, enabling us endlessly to recycle the past but preventing us from developing it. This applies to ideas as well as to goods. The thoughts that people had in previous times become either objects of study from which, via the machinery of a vast 'knowledge' industry, academics may churn out endless exegesis, or they are left behind in the pervasive fetish for 'novelty', only to be reiterated as new discoveries by people for whom true scholarship is a lost art. The future is important only for how it affects our buying habits *now;* it may thus be used as a stimulus to anxiety – something we must provide for before it's too late ('while stocks last') – but it is unlikely to be seen as something worthy of sacrifice. We do not postpone satisfactions, we anticipate them. Our attitude to the future is symbolized by the credit card – access to it is *now*. We no longer have posterity, only children.

The person becomes stripped of function, confined in space and restricted in time to a ceaseless present, and all in the name of happiness. The world which is thus created is quite grotesquely unsuited to our actual embodied existence, but we are used to it and do not, any more than blind fish in subterranean pools, complain of circumstances which are hard to imagine as otherwise.

But if the damaging nature of the environment we have created slips easily beneath the attention of our critical awareness, we certainly do not escape the painful 'symptoms' to which that damage gives rise. The process of symptom formation is quite easy to understand in the case of 'neurotic' suffering: for the onlooker who stands outside the personal predicament of individual patients, it is more often than not quite obvious that their puzzled, inarticulate sense of pain – frequently explained as 'illness' or expressed in actions distressing to self or others – is directly understandable in the light of circumstances which they cannot see (because these circumstances are not in their field of vision) or do not wish to see (i.e. repress or deceive themselves about). But this is not the sole or even special problem of 'the neurotic', who merely provides the paradigm case for a predicament shared by us all.

Frustration, neediness, chronic irritation, suspiciousness, agonized self-concern, feelings of unreality, nausea, dizziness, a whole host of 'psychosomatic' afflications through which our bodies 'protest' at the treatment we give them, nagging anxiety, rage and panic: few of us escape for any length of time from some or several of these. (And in order to try to deal with them we assemble medical, therapeutic, counselling and other 'helping' professions whose membership would threaten to outnumber potential clients were it not for the fact that the helpers themselves need help.)

Apart from the symptoms, there are the signs – i.e. indications of the injuries done to us by our condition which, however, may not themselves be experienced as unusually uncomfortable. Since we have no world to pour ourselves into, no possibility of spontaneous absorption in a society within which we may use the concepts and implements of a tradition to work towards an unknowable future we may try to make worthwhile, we become collapsed in on ourselves, not so much introspectively (a cultivable 'inner world' is in any case the invention of a romantic individualism) as self-regardingly. We observe ourselves with minute attention, alert to the sensations of our bodily organs, monitoring carefully our state of satisfaction. We have, like Guy the gorilla, only our bodies to play with, so we strut and posture in an endless parade of fashion, or we shrivel and shrink under the glare of our own self-conscious gaze. We pamper and weigh and tend ourselves, worrying obsessively about the damage to our health which our self-indulgence may create. It is utterly characteristic of our society that it supports side-by-side a huge mass-produced food industry and a huge dietary and health industry, the latter profiting from the damage caused by the former. This is reflected at the individual level by the increasing prevalence of 'bulimia' – i.e., the compulsion to voracious eating followed by self-induced vomiting. Again I must emphasize that we are caught up in these phenomena, whether at the societal or at the individual level, quite uncomprehendingly. As I hope to show later, the operation of the influences and interests involved does not appear within our personal consciousness nor under our personal control.

And yet, I suspect, beyond the reach of words, we hate this world which we have created and which force-feeds us with its happiness until we choke. There is a deadness in our eyes and an anger in the air and an almost tangible contempt for each other which seep more and more overtly from the fantasied televisual lives of the 'rich and successful' into the everyday transactions of ordinary men and women. The more sensitive among us may be so disturbed by observation of this process that they feel they are going mad – more and more people who come to see me as patients, and from all walks of life, have literally been unnerved by an increasingly commonplace brutality and indifference they cannot believe they are seeing around them.

The hatred of the less privileged for their enslaving environment is obvious – spray paint and urine are fitting enough adornments for the walls of battery housing, and who with any spirit, having too often waited shivering outside it to phone their mother or an ambulance at the dead of a winter's night, would not want to vandalize the phone box which stands almost insolently on the corner to proclaim their subjugation? But perhaps the case is little different when it comes to those who seem more obviously to profit from our society: the *fact* is that we wreck the landscape, pollute the earth and poison the seas, and treat our fellow beings with a callous unconcern. However much we may be able to deceive ourselves about the nature and consequences of these undertakings, there is still really no doubt that they are ours, and, as with the individual 'neurotic', the only sure way of determining intention is to infer it from action. From the way we treat the world and the other people in it, from our carelessness of tradition and posterity, from the official endorsement given at the very 'highest' levels to self-interest as the only possible motive and to the threat of annihilation as the legitimate ultimate goad, it seems obvious that our obsession with an entirely self-indulgent 'happiness' has as its obverse hatred, suspicion and total unconcern with what may lie, in space or time, beyond our individual lives and the satisfactions they may afford.

This is not, I am sure, a state of affairs that any of us *wants*. In order to get to grips with this paradox, one must attempt to gain a view of the way in which social forces operate *through* rather than within individuals, how *personal* conduct can only be comprehensible in the light of *collective* aims.

3

Magic, Interest and Psychology

Throughout our culture there are, I believe, widely shared and deeply held misconceptions about human psychological makeup, particularly concerning 'motivation' (or why we do things) and 'change' (or how in the course of our individual lives we may become happier, more 'adjusted' people). These misconceptions make it very difficult indeed for us to get a helpfully explanatory purchase on the reasons for psychological distress and the chances of avoiding it. So solidly are they embedded in our culture, however, we can scarcely even see them. In order fully to expose their foundations, I believe that one must approach them through what might at first seem like a detour: one must examine the nature of 'official' psychology itself.

For while there may be no very direct relation between, on the one hand, what people-in-the-street consider the causes of their actions and the possibilities for their self-improvement, and, on the other hand, the speculations of the professionals, there is little doubt that both will reflect a general cultural impetus, and this latter, for me at any rate, is easier to detect in the relatively well formulated 'official' views than in the often unspoken or more tentative assumptions of the 'ordinary person'. Though it would certainly be a mistake to suppose that 'the experts' *determine* what the 'lay' person thinks, it is altogether more likely that those forms of psychological preconception to which our culture inclines us will find their most exact expression in 'expert' opinions and procedures. More important than this, clues as to the *reasons why* we think about ourselves as we do are, I think, most clearly revealed by a clarification of the *reasons for* our having 'a psychology' at all.

In trying, then, to understand (in the two chapters following this) how we have come to adopt ideas about 'motivation' which in fact enslave us, and ideas about 'change' which delude us, I think it may be illuminating (even if only by indirect lighting) first to gain some insight into how official psychology and psychotherapy came about, and what purposes they serve.

Whether as individuals or groups, people seem particularly prone to construct for themselves a myth of origin – i.e. a story about their beginning. Psychologists are no exception. We are the children, so the story goes, not of Adam and Eve, nor even of their simian substitutes, but of science.

Though psychologists and other professionals and academics of the 'psycho-' variety quarrel bitterly amongst themselves about the legitimacy of their claim to scientific respectability, virtually all of them trace their origin to a period during the second half of the last century when scientific method came to be applied to matters of psychological concern. Most of us, in this way, live with the happy myth that, intellectually speaking, we arrived but recently on the scene, bringing with us a clear and virginally pure scientific gaze with which to peer through the murk of metaphysics and superstition which had until so recently obscured our under-standing of the workings of the human mind. It took the world a long time to get round to the one true belief – science – but as its children we are unsullied by the ignorance and incomprehension of the past, and (especially those of us in Britain and America) we now have the infallible canons of 'objective scientific method' which, as long as we remain true to them, will guide us through a future in which freedom from the errors of former times is guaranteed.

However, the very failure of psychology in its 'applied' and therapeutic forms to cope with the emotional distress and confusion which are so prevalent in our society exposes the falli-bility of our 'scientific' dogma and indicates the falsity of our myth of origin. And in fact, of course, psychology did not undergo a virgin birth in the last century, but, like any other human endeavour, evolved out of, and still serves, concerns and interests that have been identifiable within our culture for as long as its intellectual history has been recorded. Indeed, not only are psychology's claims to an *objectively valid* understanding of and a *therapeutically effective* concern with the ills which beset us false, but it is more than possible that psychology, far from minimizing, actually compounds our difficulties.

If I am not to be really seriously misunderstood, however, I must at the outset make one thing very clear, and that is that I do not regard psychologists, or psychotherapists, or practitioners of psychological medicine, as charlatans, nor do I wish in any way to impugn their motives. A charlatan is one who knowingly pretends to knowledge and ability he or she in fact does not have. As far as psychology is complicit in the social evils and self-deceptions of our time, it is so without (except perhaps for a very small minority) the knowing connivance of its practitioners. Almost without exception, the psychologists, psychotherapists and psychiatrists I have met are, professionally speaking, honest, concerned and conscientious people who work in what they see as the best interests of their clients and patients, and who do much, at the very least, to offer comfort and support to people who have no one else to turn to.

It is, however, an irony instructive of the very points I want to make in this chapter, that (with some very important exceptions) it is the 'psycho-' disciplines themselves which have led us (misguidedly) to seek the reasons for human conduct in the individual (and often conscious) motivations of those who enact it. It thus becomes extremely difficult to call into question the effects of somebody's *actions* without apparently implying an insult to the *person;* it is hard for me to suggest that what you do has an effect contrary to what you say your intention is, without seeming thereby also to suggest that you are a liar. But if we are to be able to engage with good will and mutual respect in a search for the truth of the matter, it is essential that we be able to distinguish the meaning of an action in its widest social context from the verbal account of his or her intentions the individual actor gives. The fact is that often, perhaps most often – and arguably even always – we do things for reasons of which we are not only unaware, but *could* not be aware (more will be said about this later), but of which we are understandably tempted – and easily able – to give a plausible account.

So-called neurotic symptoms are frequently the experience or expression of a distress for which individuals cannot accurately account through an examination of their own conscious purposes. This of course does not mean that their conduct and experience itself (as opposed to their conscious articulation of it) is *irrelevant* to an explanation of their distress – indeed it is likely to be crucial. In exactly the same way, psychologists must acknowledge that what they *say* they are doing may have very little relevance to what they actually are doing, and that a more satisfactory explanation must be sought elsewhere. With individuals, one has to formulate explanations (as well as evaluations) of their conduct (a) from a consideration of their history, and (b) by inferring their intentions from the actual fruits of their activity. The case is no different with collective human undertakings such as psychology.

The definition of psychology which was taught to me was 'the scientific study of human behaviour', and the chief aim of its most representative school – behaviourism – 'the prediction and control of behaviour'. I am not sure how far academic psychologists have in recent years modified the expression of this aim, but in so far as they have softened somewhat its rather stark outline, I suspect that this would stem less from any embarrassment over its almost touchingly ingenuous revelation of a dubious interest than from an uncomfortable awareness that psychologists have, over the last hundred years or so of psychology's existence as a 'scientific', laboratory discipline, been singularly unsuccessful at predicting anything of much intrinsic intellectual merit. However, what is worth noting for the purposes of the present discussion is that, despite its association with the rigours of a disinterested scientific objectivity, 'the prediction and control of human behaviour' is, as an aim of human inquiry, no new phenomenon: it expresses an intellectual aspiration as old as magic, and restates a practical interest dear to the heart of tyrants ever since time began.

One of the central arguments of this book is that, far from 'curing' people's distress, psychology too easily serves to provide us with an excuse for continuing, as a society, to inflict it. Psychology flourishes not through any truly scientific demonstration of its validity, but because, on the one hand, it feeds an age-old dream of the magical conquest of unhappiness and the achievement of power, and, on the other, it serves the interests not only of its practitioners, but more importantly of those who have actually achieved power within society and constructed an apparatus to maintain it (this, again, not *necessarily* with any consciously evil intent). Very much more than most of its practitioners would be willing to concede, then, psychology offers magical solutions to human distress which is in fact created by abuses of the very power whose interests psychology also serves. When 'ordinary people' accept that psychology represents a 'disinterested' body of 'objective' knowledge giving the best available account of their nature and difficulties – as soon, that is, as people abandon their experience of themselves in favour of the alienating dogmas of 'experts' – then the process of mystification becomes complete.

Traditionally, 'applied' psychologists – i.e. those working in the fields of health, education and industry – have claimed for themselves two principal functions: the scientific measurement of aspects of behaviour, 'personality', etc., relevant to their concerns, and a therapeutic function in dealing with 'mental disorder', 'maladjustment', and so on. Although a continuity between the witch's incantation and the psychotherapist's 'talking cure' could perhaps be established plausibly enough, it seems that even the 'scientific measurement' aspect of the modern psychologist's role also had its counterpart in what would now be considered less respectable historical precedents.

In his masterly study of religion and magic in the sixteenth and seventeenth centuries,* Keith Thomas points out that magic to some extent filled a *therapeutic* vacuum created by the disappear-

---

*K. Thomas, *Religion and the Decline of Magic*, Penguin Books, 1973.

ance of the confessional and the emergence of a note of puritanical disapproval on the part of the clergy of the kinds of problems for which people might seek help. Indeed magic, Thomas argues, 'may have provided as effective a therapy for the diseases of the mind as anything available today'.

People have always sought to influence by magical ritual what they could not control in any other way. 'Witchcraft was thus generally believed to be a method of bettering one's condition when all else had failed. Like most forms of magic, it was a substitute for impotence, a remedy for anxiety and despair.' There is of course an element of pure wishfulness about this, but, again as Thomas notes, there are *facilitative* aspects of much magical ritual which, though they form no part of its central rationale, have the effect of encouraging people to make up their minds concerning a particular course of action, or of comforting the person who distractedly seeks a solution to his or her dilemma. Divination, for example,

> could help men to take decisions when other agencies failed them. Its basic function was to shift the responsibility away from the actor, to provide him with a justification for taking a leap in the dark, and to screw him up into making a decision whose outcome was unpredictable by normal means.
>
> The diviner's predictions, therefore, did not deflect his clients from their original intentions; on the contrary, it was the process of consultation which forced them to know their own minds. Divination could set the imagination free.

In this respect, magical procedures acted precisely in the way that, as I suggested earlier, psychotherapy acts today. Psychotherapy also makes claims to technical processes of cure which are *in fact* invalid, but in the course of doing so dispenses comfort and encouragement which are far from ineffective.

Apart from the directly therapeutic significance of magical modes of thought, one may note that, for example, both in its methods (which were to a surprising extent 'objective' and statistical) and in its concerns (which included the study of 'individual differences' and human typology, vocational and educational guidance, etc.), seventeenth-century astrology bore resemblances to 'modern' psychology so strong that one can scarcely believe one is reading about a different discipline. Actually, of course, one is not:

> As Auguste Comte was to recognize, the astrologers were pioneering a genuine system of historical explanation. In their confident assumption that the principles underlying the development of human society were capable of human explanation, we can detect the germ of modern sociology.

Astrologers, apparently, even justified their failures in precisely the same way as do present-day applied psychologists. In both cases, practitioners point out that their 'scientifically established' procedures are based on an assessment of the *probability* of a particular finding, or outcome, or 'behaviour', so that one may expect there always to be a proportion of cases in which matters will go astray. Furthermore, both astrologers and psychologists confess a degree of human error: the procedures and tests used, they say, have to be to some extent *interpreted* and the accuracy of this will depend on the correct following of rules, 'clinical experience and judgment', and so on. In both cases, then, large loopholes are provided in the event of the 'scientificity' of the system being attacked. The similarity of concerns between astrology and more modern disciplines is clearly noted by Thomas:

In the absence of any rival system of scientific explanation, and in particular of the social sciences – sociology, social anthropology, social psychology – there was no other existing body of thought, religion apart, which even began to offer so all-embracing an explanation for the baffling variousness of human affairs.

As is the similarity of clinical application:

The attraction of having one's horoscope cast was not unlike that of undergoing psychoanalysis today. The reward would be a penetrating analysis of the individual's innermost attributes, the qualities which he should develop, and the limitations against which he should be on his guard.

Astrology's 'pretensions to be a genuinely scientific system' again remind one strongly of the insistence of present-day psychologists that their scientific orthodoxy must give them a right to respect and credibility, and they too would argue that their findings are based 'on the meticulous study of cause and effect'.

As far as 'modern psychology' is concerned, I see no real evidence that its findings and predictions, its so-called 'laws of behaviour', and so on, are any more soundly established or firmly based than were the claims to effectiveness of the astrologers. In my own field of clinical psychology, for example, it seems to me that scientific method has merely provided a rhetoric through which psychologists could (a) introduce ideas and practices which they *felt* to be beneficial and probably valid, and (b) create for themselves a credible professional role. Having largely succeeded in both these aims, psychologists have now for the most part abandoned the 'tough-minded' scientific stance by means of which they bought their respectability, and which would indeed now work *against* their interests because there is in truth so little scientific evidence that their procedures do in fact work. Having become firmly established professionally, psychologists now simply *assert* their effectiveness in the confident and correct expectation that this will be sufficient to maintain their standing.

But when all is said and done, it is of course a mistake to regard magic and science as *opposing* points of view, for our scientific procedures are informed by our wishful magic. As Thomas points out: 'the magical desire for power had created an intellectual environment favourable to experiment and induction: it maintained a break with the characteristic mediaeval attitude of contemplative imagination.' Science, in this way, evolves from magic.

There is indeed a sense in which scientific observation and procedure need to be dispassionate: the scientist must take note of what actually happens, as the result, for example, of experiments which have been conducted, rather than what he or she would like to happen. But it is only in a relatively limited and technical sphere that scientists need to maintain this kind of objectivity: the true scientist needs to pay proper respect to the 'embodied otherness' of the world and the things and people in it, to recognize that they are not to be *wished* in or out of existence, but this does not mean that he or she is not *passionately involved* in the search for knowledge. Above all, however dispassionate science may or may not be, it is certainly not disinterested. Francis Bacon, whose role in laying the grounds of scientific procedures is reverentially acknowledged by philosophers of science today, clearly associated his aspirations for science with the kinds of powers which at the time only magic could hope to achieve:

> Francis Bacon listed as *desiderata* the prolongation of life, the restitution of youth, the curing of incurable diseases, the mitigation of pain, the speeding up of natural processes, the discovery of new sources of food, the control of the weather, and the enhancement of the pleasures of the senses. He wanted divination put on a natural basis so that it would be possible to make rational predictions of the weather, the harvest, and the epidemics of each year. His aspirations were the same of those of the astrologers, the magicians and the alchemists, even if the methods he envisaged were different.*

This is not the pursuit of knowledge for its own sake, but of knowledge in order to dominate nature and increase the power of men. And in truth, of course, science has not made a bad job

*Thomas, op. cit.

of this enterprise (even if at a cost, in terms of pollution and impoverishment, etc., which we have yet to count). There is, however, much less hard evidence that the sciences of man, the 'psycho-' disciplines, have achieved even a tiny proportion of their aims. The evolution of natural science from magic – of, for instance, chemistry from alchemy – may be an interesting illustration of the constancy of our wishfulness and a sobering indication of our lust for power, but it is also an example of a real evolutionary movement (whether for good or for ill) in the nature of our search for knowledge. Whether the same can be said for psychology is another question, and how far it represents a distinct advance upon magic, in terms of evidential, objective knowledge, is entirely debatable.

It is my belief that, in terms of their capacity to develop and apply conceptual thought and practical action, human beings are broadly equal partners in the creation of a *moral* world (i.e. a world which cannot be technically known in advance, but must be created out of conduct we can characterize only as good or bad). If this is so, they cannot then expect to be able to understand or treat each other as if *some* of them were *objects*; methods of objective, natural science cannot be expected to bear fruit when applied to a community of subjects (which is the only proper, and in the long run possible, way of regarding the human community).

Psychology then, it seems to me, is still much more closely related to magic than is, say, chemistry. Partly, no doubt, one can explain its continuing success because like magic, in Thomas's words, it 'lessens anxiety, relieves pent-up frustration, and makes the practitioner feel that he is doing something positive towards the solution of his problem'. But I think that there are more powerful reasons which support the practice of psychology quite apart from its convincing use of scientific rhetoric and its incidental provision of comfort and encouragement to those who lack more effective remedies for their ills, and consideration of these will once again involve us in an examination of the operation of interest.

Thomas himself notes the role played by some magical procedures in associating misfortune with moral blame, and hence contributing to forces of social control. It is precisely this aspect – that of social control through the establishment of *individual* guilt and accountability – which has become, in my view, the principal function of psychology, and which serves to maintain it in so flourishing an existence within our society.

Modern psychology's aim to 'predict and control human behaviour', as well as its investment in the theory and practice of conditioning (particularly strong in the behaviourist school and the associated 'behaviour therapies'), may claim a significant part of their ancestry in the writings of the seventeenth-century philosopher John Locke. Showing the same kind of innocence which was noted in the last chapter in the case of the Utilitarians writing a century later, Locke seems unaware that his proposals for the effective education, or perhaps rather shaping, of the individual would ever be put to any use other than the perfecting of mankind. To our ears, however, there is already a rather sinister ring to his proposals. In advocating the establishment in children of *habit* through the judicious use of praise and blame (encouragement and shame), Locke writes:

> If by these means you can come once to shame them out of their faults, (for besides that, I would willingly have no punishment) and make them in love with the pleasure of being well thought on, you may turn them as you please, and they will be in love with all the ways of virtue.*

From this, as Passmore notes:

> It will at once be obvious that Locke has opened up, in principle, the possibility of perfecting men by the application of readily intelligible, humanly controllable, mechanisms. All that is required is that there should be an educator, or a social group, able and willing to teach the child what to pursue and what to avoid.

Here lies, in a nutshell, the whole point and purpose of the vast enterprise which present-day psychology has become: the location of the means of social control *inside the heads of the very individuals who are to be controlled*. Compare Locke's benign view of what has come to be known as 'behavioural shaping' or 'behaviour modification' with the altogether less palatable perspective of Servan, who wrote in late eighteenth-century France of the necessity to link the *ideas* of crime and punishment in the *minds* of people such that they

> follow one another without interruption . . . When you have thus formed the chain of ideas in the heads of your citizens, you will then be able to pride yourselves on guiding them and being their masters. A stupid despot may constrain his slaves with iron chains; but a true politician binds them even more strongly by the chain of their own ideas; it is at the stable point of reason that he secures the end of the chain; this link is all the stronger in that we do not know of what it is made and we believe it to be our own work; despair and

---

*Quoted in Passmore, op.cit.

time eat away the bonds of iron and steel, but they are powerless against the habitual union of ideas, they can only tighten it still more; and on the soft fibres of the brain is founded the unshakable base of the soundest of Empires.*

Already one begins to see why, having considered the associationist psychology which grew out of Locke's philosophical analysis, Passmore should judge that:

It is not surprising that, under Pavlov's influence, such a psychology won official approval in the Soviet Union and wide acceptance in the United States, both of them countries which are deeply involved in the technological 'management' of human beings . . .

Independent testimony to the success of this enterprise is lent by the words of two modern American writers, who in the course of a disturbing analysis of the uses to which 'therapeutic' psychology has been put in the United States to control the behaviour of children who are in one way or another troublesome to authority, note that 'behaviour modification can make the effects of such authority more painless than, for example, the use of a club or the threat of punishment, but in its ideal form it will erase all awareness of its existence and thereby make it absolute.'†

Nobody has done more than Michel Foucault to show how the development over the last few centuries of the human sciences has become saturated throughout with the interests of power. In his magnificent book *Discipline and Punish*, for example, he argues that 'all the sciences, analyses or practices employing the root "psycho"' have arisen in the course of a process in which the punishment of illegal *acts* by otherwise anonymous malefactors, has turned into the maintenance of discipline in *people* by means of an ever more finely differentiated analysis of their individual characteristics. Where once the state discouraged threats against it through an ostentatiously terrifying recourse to spectacular tortures and execution, it now does it through a scientific technology of power – i.e. discipline. Through the use of scientific observation, the objectifying 'gaze' which seeks to see without itself being seen (a necessity well known to every student of psychology in search of 'uncontaminated' observations), social scientists become practitioners of a discipline which dissects, orders and normalizes indi-

---

*Quoted in M. Foucault, *Discipline and Punish*, Penguin Books, 1979.
†P. Schrag and D. Divoky, *The Myth of the Hyperactive Child and Other Means of Child Control*, Penguin Books, 1981.

viduals, and documents and traces the roots of their differentiation or dissent.

The establishment of such discipline is aided by several factors. There is, for example, the actual apparatus of observation, corresponding to the microscope of the physical scientist: in this respect Foucault writes particularly interestingly of the 'panopticon', i.e. the physical structure whereby human beings could be observed or studied in large numbers by as few as one unseen watcher. The prototype of this design is the circular prison, in which cells are constructed around the circumference, facing inwards in such a way that one warder in the centre would have a direct view of all prisoners. This kind of structure, several examples of which were built in the last century, has its parallel today in the one-way glass screens to be found in every university department of psychology. (It is characteristic of Foucault's genius to bring one suddenly face-to-face with a question at once blindingly obvious and excruciatingly revealing: if psychologists' intentions are honourable – as we have always felt and asserted them to be – why *do* they need to shield people from their gaze?)

Apart from the physical paraphernalia of observation, the technology of power has other tools of its trade – for example the concept of delinquency, which allows the punisher of *acts* to become the disciplinarian who, as it were, invades the internal space of individuals in order to establish and track their *reasons*; instead of punishing the wrongdoer's action, you thus control his or her biography. There is also the procedure of the examination:

> The examination combines the techniques of an observing hierarchy and those of a normalizing judgment. It is a normalizing gaze, a surveillance that makes it possible to qualify, to classify and to punish. It establishes over individuals a visibility through which one differentiates them and judges them. That is why, in all the mechanisms of discipline, the examination is highly ritualized. In it are combined the ceremony of power and the form of the experiment, the deployment of force and the establishment of truth. At the heart of the procedures of discipline, it manifests the subjection of those who are perceived as objects and the objectification of those who are subjected.

For modern men and women who have never experienced what it is like *not* to live under the 'normalizing' gaze of educational, medical and scientific experts of one kind or another, and who have been subjected from their earliest days to a rhetoric which emphasizes the benefits of living in a 'free world', the suggestion that we are seriously constrained by the unseen discipline of our social institutions may seem simply incredible. Examinations, for example, seem to be the 'natural' and 'obvious' ways to test educational achievement, and indeed the educational system itself seems the 'natural' and 'obvious' way to impart knowledge to the young. At the same time, I think, we all of us have the evidence of our own experience to suggest that Foucault and others are not wrong to alert us to the extent to which our social institutions do curtail our freedom and cripple our potentialities as human beings. For example, who does not know for him- or herself the savage tyranny of the 'norm'? Being different, standing out, *feeling* differently from others, experiencing oneself as conspicuous in some way — feelings such as these are at the very core of much of what gets called 'psychiatric disorder', and indeed of the everyday terrors of us all. That such feelings are so familiar a part of our ordinary experience leads us to consider them as 'human nature', but much more likely, I suspect, is that they are the internalized values of a society which depends for its smooth economic functioning on the *willing* obedience of the individual. *Punishment* of illegality has become, through the processes so brilliantly described by Foucault, individual *guilt* over non-conformity.

Although the vast majority of those involved professionally in the technology of discipline (and ultimately in the engineering of *self*-discipline) tend to be quite unaware of their contribution (feeling instead that their role is merely one of scientific inquiry or therapeutic service), this is not true of all, and Foucault's insights find their echo in the observations of some of those much more directly engaged at the professional level. Not surprisingly, however, the most trenchant criticism tends to come from those who obtain a clear view of the 'psycho-' disciplines from outside. It takes, for example, two journalists, Schrag and Divoky,* to point out what the actual effects of 'screening' programmes for American children may be. A combination of parental anxiety, professional self-interest and undercurrent concern over social unrest resulted, they write, in a situation in which:

> Between 1971 and 1974, thirty states passed special education laws and more are doing so each year; many of these mandate the screening of entire school populations not only for defective vision and hearing, for malnutrition and bad teeth, but for 'oedipal conflicts', 'ego disturbances' and 'normalcy' in 'impulse control', 'withdrawal' and 'social

The Myth of the Hyperactive Child and Other Means of Child Control, op. cit.

behaviour'. Such screening is now common, even for four-year-olds.

While procedures such as these are justified by a rhetoric of welfare, their actual effect is that

> this generation is learning at a very young age that there is nothing unusual about being watched, questioned, tested, labelled and 'treated', or about the fact that the results of all that watching and questioning are being stored and processed in machines over which the individual has no control. It is hardly worth saying again that the existence of such a record can have a chilling effect or that privacy is 'the right to be left alone'. But for those who have become habituated to such records and treatment from the age of five, that chilling effect may never occur because they have never been left alone, and they will therefore never suspect that there might have been another way.

And so:

> An entire generation is slowly being conditioned to distrust its own instincts, to regard its deviation from the narrowing standards of approved norms as sickness and to rely on the institutions of the state and on technology to define and engineer its 'health'.

If one is to understand the processes whereby 'scientific psychology' comes to cooperate with the state in the realization of the latter's interests, one must, I think, guard against the temptation – at times very strong – to attribute to those involved, i.e. the economically powerful, the politicians and the 'scientific' professionals, implication in some kind of malevolent conspiracy. Although it would no doubt be equally mistaken to *rule out* the possibility that there can be quite deliberate and conscious components to the exploitation of the weak by the strong, the process of exploitation as a whole is probably facilitated most of all by our having been overtaken in recent times by a general lowering of moral and political awareness. 'Politics and religion', together perhaps with too indecently direct reference to money (as in the question of how much a person earns), have become subjects which many people feel it indelicate to inquire into too closely or too publicly. This constitutes a form of repression the effect of which (as is, after all, commonly the case with repression) is to allow the interests which might otherwise be challenged by, in this case, moral and political awareness to operate all the more unrestrainedly. Professional collaborators with such interests have in this way no particular consciousness of the significance of their collaboration. Economic values have largely replaced moral and political ones in the public awareness, so that anything which appears to be conducive to the 'creation of wealth', or at least to economic stability, is taken as self-evidently desirable.

'Ordinary people', moreover, feel powerless to challenge an oppressive system partly because the channels of moral and political *understanding* which were once available (for example in the days when political pamphlets would be read in hundreds of thousands) have largely become closed off to them. (As noted earlier, this feeling of powerlessness is, these days, *very frequently* a complaint of people suffering from 'symptoms' of psychological distress, many of whom explicitly recognize that the information that would enable them to make judgments about socially significant and disturbing issues – for example 'the bomb', racial unrest – is not available in those 'media' to which they have ready access.)

It is thus with almost disarming political naivety that H. J. Eysenck – Britain's best-known psychologist – could write of a 'technology of consent':

> which will make people behave in a socially adapted, law-abiding fashion, which will not lead to a breakdown of the intricately interwoven fabric of social life . . . a generally applicable method of inculcating suitable habits of socialized conduct into the citizens (and particularly the future citizens) of the country in question – or preferably the whole world.*

Psychology's most significant contribution to modern society is less 'scientific' or 'therapeutic' than managerial. The task shaped by the economic interests of this century has been to shift the ordinary person's orientation from production to consumption, and this has been achieved by expropriating his or her knowledge and skill so that they can become mechanized and managed in a mass market. Indeed, this programme has at times been put into operation entirely consciously in the name of 'scientific management':

> The managers assume . . . the burden of gathering together all the traditional knowledge which in the past has been possessed by the workmen and then of classifying, tabulating and reducing this knowledge to rules, laws and formulae . . .

*H. J. Eysenck, The technology of consent. *New Scientist*, 42, 688–90, June 1969. For this and the following quotations from Taylor, I am indebted to Dr John Shotter.

Because:

> . . . all the planning which under the old system was done by the workman, as a result of his personal experience, must of necessity under the new system be done by the management in accordance with the laws of science.*

The prestige of 'science' becomes associated with whatever social processes are necessary for the achievement of the economic interests of power, and to this purpose the 'social sciences' lend themselves admirably. As Schrag and Divoky put it:

> The normative assumptions and natural order invoked by the new modes of control are, in one sense, disciplinary replacements for Social Darwinism. Each in its own time was (or is) 'scientific'. But while Social Darwinism was almost entirely an economic 'law' concerned with the individual's fitness for the labour market (and particularly the factory), its contemporary substitute is concerned with every aspect of the individual's life and, most particularly, with his potential as a client. The system no longer requires his muscle, but it needs his obedience. It no longer must train him to be a reliable worker, but it must condition him to be managed.

What Christopher Lasch calls the 'tutelary complex' − i.e. the amalgam of educational, social and therapeutic agencies concerned with our 'adjustment' − has in fact become the instrument of managerial discipline. In a passage strongly reminiscent of Foucault, he suggests that the tutelary complex:

> . . . both reflects and contributes to the shift from authoritative sanctions to psychological manipulation and surveillance − the redefinition of political authority in therapeutic terms − and to the rise of a professional and managerial class that governs society not by upholding authoritative moral standards but by defining normal behaviour and by invoking allegedly non-punitive, psychiatric sanctions against deviance.†

Interest is at once the most powerful and the least honourable motivation of human conduct. Unchecked, its operation is likely to be extremely destructive, since its long-term effect is to wear away the ligaments which bind a society in *communal* purpose. If, into the bargain, its operation is repressed − i.e. unnoticed and

---

*F. W. Taylor, *Scientific Management*, Harper and Bros., 1947 (first published 1918).

†*The Minimal Self*, op. cit.

uncommented-upon – the destructiveness to which it gives rise may turn out to be uncontrollable. That psychology – supposedly the 'scientific study of human behaviour' – concerns itself not at all with the operation of interest (though it is itself heavily caught up in it), testifies, in, as it were, silent eloquence, to the extent to which we *do* repress awareness of the operation of interest. We simply do not talk about nor even notice the degree to which our conduct, at all levels, is aimed at the exploitation of the world and of each other purely for selfish gain, nor do we see that a great deal of the distress we experience *personally*, in our everyday lives, is traceable to the currents of interest in whose destructive vortices we are caught up.

We have in our present society largely dismantled the moral structures by means of which the operation of interest may be checked, and through the acceptance of mass-market economies as somehow inevitably *necessary* we have reduced almost to vanishing point the degree to which political opposition can expose and cancel out the operation of competitive interests. In these circumstances, it becomes all the more important to increase *awareness* of the degree to which we are under the sway of interest – i.e. to lift our repression of it.

There are perhaps some signs that the appeal of cupidity and self-interest is becoming less disguised than even a few years ago, but this seems to be happening not so much through a frank acknowledgment of greed as through an association of 'market forces' with a kind of unexamined moral imperative: interest is breaking free of moral restraint by linking itself directly with an *assertion* of moral authority – cost-benefit analysis becomes the *fundamental* measure of right and wrong. (The technique of assertion is, of course, itself characteristic of the marketing society, and replaces now almost outmoded methods of what one might call 'evidential' persuasion. When what matters is *whether* rather than *why* you buy – the economy *must*, after all, expand – attempts to convince you of a commodity's value by a rational appeal to *evidence* of its qualities give way to an almost ritual *assertion* of those qualities, a kind of authoritative confirmation that it is indeed up for sale, and therefore *ought* to be bought. As I have already indicated in the case of clinical psychology, the technique of assertion extends far beyond the boundaries of what we have traditionally considered the 'market-place'.)

The extent to which the workings of interest are cloaked in repression is still, however, very great, and represents a process in which we are all implicated. Disavowed interest, one might say, is the barely visible oil which keeps the cogs of the acquisitive society turning. Interest works, indeed, not by the brutal oppression of one section of society by another, but through the interlocking of many types and sub-sets of interests. I may achieve what *I* want (which may easily be against your interest) by recruiting you to my cause through making the attainability of what *you* want appear dependent upon your falling in with my desires. This is of course nothing other than the ancient art of manipulation long known to politicians and horse-traders, but I think we fail to acknowledge how large a part it plays in our conduct, as well as how unrestrained and dangerous the game becomes when it is fuelled by an individualistic pursuit of happiness and unchecked by any overarching moral purpose.

In the context of the interlocking of our interests, our conduct tends to slide always in the same direction of exploitation and maximization of perceived personal gain, harnessing as it goes baser and baser and coarser and coarser motivations in order to increase the saleability and consumption of our 'products'. This slide takes place in an almost infinite number of finely graded steps. The space between our potential and our actual actions may well be occupied by *feigned* considerations of right and wrong, but it is *in fact* occupied by the promptings of interest. One might almost formulate a 'law of human behaviour' in this respect (and one, I fear, more accurate at the present time than many advanced by experimental psychologists over the last hundred years): 'faced with a number of courses of action having roughly equal probability of achievement, a person is likely to choose that which conforms most to his/her self-interest'. Furthermore, what the individual *sees as* in his or her interest will be manipulated by higher-order interests, with the degree of superordinacy of an interest or set of interests being determined by economic power. We are thus led more or less automatically into forms of relationship and communication which are entirely manipulative. The more power a person or a group has, the more will it be able to determine the perceptions of their interest held by those lower in the power hierarchy, so that what low-status people *see as* in their interests will probably not be so, but will *in fact* be in the interests of the relatively more powerful.

Because the workings of interest are impersonal in the sense that they do not spring from the conscious intentions of particular people, it is very hard to find a language in which to express them. In this respect, one is reminded of nothing so much as the 'Invisible Hand' which Adam Smith described as responsible for the workings of the market economy, and which is extolled so enthusiastically by his present-day admirers. Thus, individual people *appear* to be absolved (since they are unaware of it) from complicity in a process in which some of them are subjugated to the interests of others while all *believe* that they benefit.

Since we are so unaccustomed to locating *ourselves* within this process, and have no real concepts with which to do so, it is hard to think of succinct or sharply drawn examples of its operation. At the simplest and most direct level, however, most people capable of honest reflection on their own conduct will be aware of how easy it is to slide towards rationalizations of actions which are beneficial (to themselves) rather than right (this is a distinction which will be taken up in greater detail in the final chapter of this book). Two apples are left in the bowl; though I am better fed and richer than you, I take the larger one, perhaps guiltily acknowledging to myself my greed and perhaps not, but in any case telling myself more emphatically that the slight blemish on its skin in fact makes it less desirable and nutritious than the other which I graciously leave for you.

At a less personal level, it may be easiest to see how, for instance, interest can disguise itself as necessity by examining the conduct of people other than ourselves; let me take directly from my own experience an example which I think at the same time illustrates processes typical of the 'managerial' ethos of so-called 'post-industrial society' on a much wider scale. The activity of some National Health Service administrators has in recent times undergone a striking change from the concerned, meticulous support of procedures of clinical care once characteristic of them to a kind of swashbuckling managerial bravado in which cuts in services to patients and jobs of staff are made with apparent indifference or even satisfaction. The same people whose conduct not long ago would have been cautious, balanced, concerned for fairness, now speak the hard, almost macho language of 'the real world' and of the need for 'efficiency and effectiveness', and actually express pride in cutting costs by measures which, ironically, are clearly neither in their own direct interests nor in those of the staff and patients for whom they are responsible. But there *are* ways in which their interests are caught up in this process. Their *perceived* interest lies in their 'image' of themselves as 'managers' – no longer are they seen by 'colleagues in industry' as bumbling clerical functionaries doing a second-rate job of administration in an over-protected public service: they are *managers* making the kinds of hard but necessary decisions made by executives of oil companies (as seen on TV). They conform to a style and rhetoric which has been sanctioned and endorsed from high above them by governmental power aimed at dismantling public health care. Their *negative* interest lies in the feeling that if they did not so conform there could be a threat to their jobs, though apart from this there is no tangible advantage to their conduct,* and indeed considerable impairment to the moral quality of their work. These are decent people whose conduct springs not from some kind of illusory personal autonomy, but from a social context structured by interest.

It would certainly be entirely misleading to locate the reasons for interest-shaped conduct in the gullibility, perversity or 'selfishness' of people themselves: as I shall try to elaborate in greater detail in the course of the next two chapters, people react in relation to a world which impinges directly upon them, but which is largely shaped by forces not in their sight. The profound and pervasive significance of this process has become most obvious to me through working with 'patients' whose conduct is inexplicable, to themselves as well as to me, in terms of conventional understandings of personal autonomy. Why, for example, does someone with a serious physical condition such as diabetes or kidney failure make precisely those dietary preferences which create an otherwise avoidable threat to life or limb? (Why *do* people smoke or work in asbestos mines?) Why do people fail to take measures which would quite obviously result in improvements to their personal condition or circumstances? Above all, it has dawned on me – all too slowly – that the straight distress people feel cannot be explicated by the traditional conceptual paraphernalia of psychology and psychotherapy, etc., but arises out of a highly complex interaction between the economic coercion which bears directly upon them (you work in asbestos mines rather than starve) and the availability to them of information, ideas and language which would allow them to develop an understanding of their position. This picture is further complicated by the fact that information, ideas and language, once acquired (according to processes again to be elaborated in the following chapters), are not easily altered. This entire complex of

*Since these words were written the British government has adopted an altogether more workmanlike approach to the manipulation of managerial interest. The *Guardian*, 3 September 1986, reports that: 'Health authority managers could be denied an annual pay rise if they fail to achieve their individual targets under the Department of Health's new merit pay system . . . But those "consistently exceeding short-term objectives and making excellent progress towards long-term goals" will be awarded an extra 4 per cent on salary in the first year . . . Health service unions have attacked the plan as an incentive scheme for accelerating hospital closures and service cuts . . .' The article goes on to describe how each tier of management will be 'assessed' by those next highest in authority. This provides as good an example as any of how interest can be manipulated via a pyramidal hierarchy ('management') in order to achieve higher-order political goals.

interacting factors is shaped by the invisible handiwork of interest into a disciplinary network from which there is virtually no escape.

Take, for example, a gentle and sensitive man of thirty who is thought to be suffering from a 'mild depressive illness' because of his 'unrealistic fears' of contamination at work and a preoccupation with bronchial discomfort, his gloomy concerns about the state of the world and his 'undue absences' from work. He works in a machine shop clouded with industrial dust; he is worried about the bomb, the frequency of rape and racial tension; he is afraid that the vegetables in his garden may be polluted by fall-out from the Chernobyl nuclear accident, and further afraid that this must mean he's crazy. On the face of it, it may well seem that his difficulties are 'unrealistic' because they all admit of some kind of solution. *But only if he is empowered to act within the space available to him.* Why, for example, shouldn't he wear a mask (as he is supposed to) at work if he is worried about bronchial trouble? Because his much 'tougher' workmates ridicule him if he does. Why doesn't he get another job, then? He has tried, but there aren't any. If he's worried about the state of the world, why doesn't he become socially and politically active? Because he is barely literate and doesn't know where to start; he has not learned the highly complex conceptual competence which comes as second nature to those, for example, who have received a middle-class education. His horizons are all but inescapably limited by the comics he reads, ITV news and the *Sun* newspaper. The tragedy is that he is a gentle, intelligent, loving and thoughtful man whose very sensitivity, in contrast to the hardened survivors who surround him, makes him feel aberrant and even unhinged (which of course, in relation to his context, he is). He likes his West Indian and Asian workmates, but still thinks they ought to go 'home' because 'they are taking the jobs of real people'; this is the best judgment he can make not because he is a 'racist' but because he has been denied the conceptual and informational equipment which makes any more sophisticated view possible. (If this seems incredible, remember how difficult it must have been to learn things which seem so easy to you now; or imagine, for example, suddenly being required to perform some complex task which is somebody else's child's play – glass blowing, perhaps, or speaking Finnish. 'All very well,' you may say, 'but at least he could look at Channel Four instead of ITV.' But from his point of view, 'people like me' don't do things like that: they no more read unusual books or watch unusual television programmes than the average professional person attends court functions or rides to hounds, and for precisely the same reason.) Why, again, does he not wash the vegetables in his garden to accommodate what is after all a perfectly legitimate concern? Because authority has instructed him that there is no need to, and he therefore experiences his own doubt as irrational (those at the base of our power hierarchy are trained to trust unquestioningly in authority).

At the bottom of the heap there is not a great deal of room for manoeuvre, and whatever autonomy one has is likely to be strictly limited to the most immediate personal concerns. Those sufferers from diabetes, for example, who knowingly risk severe future injury to their health by eating and drinking too much of the wrong things, do so largely because the pleasures and possibilities of their lives are limited to eating and drinking: their conduct in these respects, though immediately 'motivated' by such restricted satisfactions, is in fact held in place by a network of interlocking interests quite out of their sight, and is far from irrational in terms of their personal circumstances.

It is no doubt easier to see how one can be the victim of the hierarchy of power than the victimizer, and yet both roles are played out unconsciously by the vast majority of us. People further up the hierarchy, having more room for manoeuvre, more access to information and ideas, etc., are perhaps likely to be more plausibly convinced of their personal autonomy, but here again their conduct will be powerfully shaped by the interests bearing upon it from above, and in the process will interlock in a coercive way with that of those in a weaker position.

In the barest possible outline, then, one may be able to glimpse in these far from polished reflections the potential for a psychology of interest which psychology itself has not even started to make *explicit*, but in which it has been extensively *complicit*. Indeed, the growth of psychology as a 'scientific' discipline is itself instructive of the way interests interlock to bring about particular forms of socio-economic organization *as well as* to shape the direction taken by supposedly disinterested academic and intellectual bodies. Though, arguably, European, and in particular German academic psychology towards the latter half of the nineteenth century was overshadowed by the relatively abstract concerns of philosophy, it received an altogether more practical impetus when it was imported into the United States. As K. Danziger argues, rather than having to justify themselves to their more academically respectable colleagues in faculties of philosophy:

> . . . psychologists had to justify themselves before a very different tribunal. Control of university appointments, research funds, and professional opportunities was vested in the hands of either businessmen and their appointees, or politicians who represented their interests. If psychology was

to emerge as a viable independent discipline, it would have to be in a form acceptable to these social forces. The inclinations of those on whose decisions the fate of American psychology depended were clear. They were men in positions of genuine social power who were anxious to use their positions to control the actions of others. They were interested in techniques of social control and in tangible performance. Their image of man was hardly that of the contemplative philosopher: a huge system of secondary and professional education had to be built practically from scratch; the human fallout from wide-scale migration and urbanization had to be dealt with; man had to be made to adapt to a rapidly rationalized industrial system; products had to be sold. In view of the weakness of alternative sources of professional expertise, psychologists might become acceptable if they could reasonably promise to develop the technical competence needed to deal appropriately with these problems.*

Bearing in mind the researches of Foucault, one would probably be unwise to take the difference between European and North American psychology as one of kind rather than merely as one of degree. However that may be, it does seem that present-day Anglo-American psychology cannot by any stretch of the imagination accurately be cast in the role of disinterested scientific pursuit, nor its practical branches be understood as merely the therapeutic application of insights derived from the laboratory.

As I hope I have already made clear, I do not wish to say that there is no scientific truth in psychology and even less do I want to suggest that there is no good to be derived from psychotherapy. But if we are to extract what is true and good from psychology and psychotherapy, it is essential that as far as we can we disentangle the strands of truth and goodness from those of magic and interest. In particular, it is of vital importance to expose the extent to which psychology has been used to mystify an understanding of the reasons for our conduct, and therapy to stifle our often anguished protests at the injustices of our world, all in the interest of the smooth running of a society which threatens to destroy us.

*K. Danziger, The social origins of modern psychology. In R. Buss (ed.) *Psychology in Social Context*, Irvington Publishers Inc., 1979.

4

Faults and Reasons

Who is to blame? Whose fault is it? That is the question which seems these days to leap to the mind of anyone who tries to understand the causes of unhappiness. It is, for example, conspicuously the question which obsesses all those – particularly journalists, 'media people' and politicians – who have some part to play in the public analysis of misfortune or unrest. Most inquiries into politically significant disturbances or catastrophes seem to come to rest once the blame for them has been established, and indeed the haste to identify a blameworthy person or group is often positively indecent. 'Activists', 'extremists', 'criminal elements' – these are the familiar targets of blame whose identification somehow satisfies, or perhaps rather pre-empts, our need to understand the causes of disturbance in our society. The search for a person or people to blame is equally remorseless in the case of less obviously politically loaded misfortunes. A child is battered to death: do we blame the parents, or do we blame the social workers, health visitors, doctors who had contact with the family? An aeroplane crashes: do we blame the pilot, the manufacturers, the maintenance engineers, the air traffic controllers? We do not, it seems, rest happy until we have located the cause of the disaster *inside* a person or group of people.

The case is no different with our individual conduct and experience. Whose fault is my unhappiness? Is it mine, is it yours, my spouse's, mother's, employer's?

And yet we have not always been so obsessed with blame. Explanations for why people do things, or react in the way that they do to what has been done, seem to conform (within limits) to fashion. Not long ago, for example, the fashion was to refer for explanations of human distress to concepts of illness, i.e. to impersonal, 'dysfunctional' mechanisms within people. Just recently, the fashion has become more to look for some kind of (largely unelaborated) moral failing. In psychotherapy, it used to be an advance for patients to accept a measure of responsibility for their actions, since this allowed them to get a subjective grip on their circumstances rather than seeing their 'inadequacy' as the result of some kind of mechanical deficiency. Now, however, it seems a positive disadvantage for patients to see themselves as responsible for their actions, since they appear not to be able to make a conceptual differentiation between responsibility and blame. What formerly was a route to at least a measure of subjective effectiveness has now become a terminus in guilty despair.

The reason for these movements of fashion in explanation lies in the fact that individual psychology cannot be understood outside the context of a social world. Times change, and with them our individual conception of ourselves. It would be absurd to suppose that any one of us can escape the influence of our social, political, economic and cultural environment, and hence any attempt to construct an *absolute* psychology appealing to unchanging fundamental principles must be a mistake. But, as I tried to show in the previous chapter, our psychology may not be designed so much to reflect the 'truth' of our situation as to shape our ideas about ourselves, and in this it has not been so inconsistent: it does indeed seem clear that, though fashion may change in the explanations we seek for what we do, they have consistently and increasingly over the last few centuries been focused on the *individual*. Whether 'fault' is mechanical or moral, it is seen as inside individual people, and it is precisely the 'psycho-' disciplines, with their internal probing, measuring, normalizing techniques, which make the plausibility of individual fault seem almost unassailable.

To depart from the norm in virtually any direction is, practically by definition, to become conspicuously deviant, and conspicuousness is attended for most of us by a kind of rush of anxious shame. It is this emotion – the panicky dread of being 'different' – which signals our departure from, and so pushes us back into conformity with, the internalized values of a society which turns us into standardized objects. Completely accustomed to a bureaucracy of power which measures, assesses, evaluates, dockets and labels us from birth to death, we have now, through the transformation of outside blame into inside shame, become our own disciplinarians. In precisely this way, people who have been damaged by the callousness and injustice of our social organization become not angry but anxious, and see their predicament as a function of their own inadequacy. The most perfect form of social control is that which is accepted by those it oppresses as necessary and inevitable. The progression from punishment to discipline traced so brilliantly by Foucault finds its completion in our time in the imposition of *self*-discipline – a conformity, that is, which is self-imposed, and which we experience as (for the most part inarticulate) shame.

If, however, we are to elaborate an accurate understanding of our condition, we must come to recognize the barbaric fallacy involved in the individualization of fault. The current fashion for blame (which, after all, so obviously does not *explain* anything) seems to me to reveal more clearly the fallacy of individualization than did the (also by no means defunct!) fashion for mechanistic, 'illness' explanations, since the latter were able to draw 'credibility' from the fundamentally technological nature of modern cultural concerns. Both, however, serve the same purpose: they assist the repression of interest. For as long as we seek the explanation for pain, despair and catastrophe *inside* people, we shall fail to observe that they are in fact the result of our construction of a society serving the functions of power and interest as they operate coercively and manipulatively *between* people. If we are to preserve from ourselves and disguise from others the spectacle of the damage and injury done by our ruthless pursuit of our own interest (in the form of 'happiness') we must create unquestioning allegiance to the view that our misfortunes stem from personal failings, whether mechanical or moral: the casualties of our system can 'only have themselves to blame'.

The transparent irrationality of equating blame with explanation does, however, make it hard to understand the extent to which people seem ready not to inquire into the reasons for events or circumstances beyond a mere imputation of blame for their occurrence. Though neither have a great deal to recommend them, in an apparent 'progression' from scientism (mechanistic explanation) to moralism (moral fault-finding) we seem if anything to be in retreat from rationality, since moralism offers no form of explanation at all. And yet, perhaps, the degree of popularity seeming recently to be enjoyed by the 'New Right', by fundamentalist religions, and by moralistic tracts masquerading as psychiatry,* may reflect an undercurrent recognition that our troubles are indeed *of our own making*, and in this sense such popularity may appear to be not entirely undeserved. At the same time, as long as any such implicit acknowledgment of our moral responsibility for ourselves is set within an individualizing psychology, it is not only utterly misleading, but adds cruelty to error. To see people's despair as arising from internal mechanical fault is simply incorrect, though convenient and even humane; to see it as arising from *personal* moral failing is both wrong and cruel even if it does gain a degree of plausibility through a relatively healthy reaction against the radical *impersonality* of mechanistic explanations. The persuasiveness, such as it is, of Wood's heartless book may in fact derive from an intelligent, if fairly obvious, analysis of the rank improbability of many of the more scientistic approaches to 'neurosis', but it shares with them a view that the cures as well as causes of distress lie *inside* the person.

Even psychoanalysis — perhaps one of the most honest and, at

---

*See for example the insightlessly uncompassionate view of psychological distress taken by G. Wood in his *The Myth of Neurosis*.

least potentially, genuinely scientific attempts to elaborate a human psychology – fails to get far beyond the notion of individual responsibility, despite recognizing that people act for reasons of which they are not conscious. Implicit in the psychoanalytic understanding of the reasons for our conduct is the view that they are rooted, beyond the reach of awareness, in our personal history, but that, through the consciousness-raising procedures of analytic therapy itself, their effects may be put within the influence of our will.* One could not possibly say that this kind of view is entirely wrong, but at the same time it leaves too much out of account not to be harmfully misleading. In locating the causes of distress in individual experience, and in implying that the amelioration of distress is a task for the individual will, psychoanalysis places itself squarely with the other 'psycho-' disciplines in fostering the interests of power; it obscures the fact that what damages us above all are the injuries we cause ourselves and each other as we struggle in the net of inducements and constraints thrown over us by our interest-saturated social organization.

It is indeed the case, as any psychotherapist well knows and as I have already had occasion to point out more than once, that people do not know why they conduct themselves as they do. Partly (as I argued at greater length in *Illusion and Reality*) this is because so much of what we do falls outside the sphere of words. The fact that we possess language gives us the mistaken idea that we can describe everything, including the reasons for our day-to-day activity, in its terms. But, of course, a great deal of what we do is unconscious in the sense that we cannot put it into a verbal form. Beyond this, however, is the fact that the reasons for much of what we do are not even *in principle* available to our consciousness, and it is *this* fact which our beliefs about our reasons for our conduct, and our official psychologies, are above all designed to repress: we come to feel personally to blame for social injustices which are in fact perpetrated far beyond the reach of our awareness.

Our society is constructed as a hierarchy of exploitation based on power. Its satisfactory functioning *depends upon* those lower in the hierarchy not being able to gain sight of the way their conduct is shaped by the interests of those higher in the hierarchy. At every level in this society conduct is shaped by the manipulation of interest in the relations *between* people. Society, in this way, organizes itself around an unequal distribution of power through the 'sliding together' of interlocking interests. Since responsibility

*Some analysts, however, have struggled hard to take account of the difficulties involved in this view – see in particular R. Schafer, *A New Language for Psychoanalysis*, Yale University Press, 1976.

for this state of affairs is itself distributed, no doubt unevenly, throughout society (in the sense that we all contribute to it), and since there is no *necessary* correlation of interestedness with awareness, the blueprint for social organization is not to be found in any person's head, nor in the heads of any group of people (though it may well be true that it is likely to be more available for articulation to those high in the hierarchy). The explanation of our conduct is thus not to be sought in a psychological analysis of individuals, but in a socio-economic, historical analysis of relations between people, and of the ways these have shaped the world we have to live in. Even in the case where an oppressor is perfectly aware of the principles whereby his or her oppression is maintained, and of what are its fruits in terms of personal gain, and even if he or she actively furthers the oppression, it would still be misleading to seek an *explanation* for it *inside* the oppressor. This is presumably why, whatever its morality, assassination is of doubtful practical value as a solution in cases of tyranny.

The imputation of blame, and also of self-blame in the form of guilt, usually arises in circumstances where a wider social view is for some reason blinkered. Where, as it so frequently is, it is in the interests of the unequal distribution of power within society to cloud this wider view, blame and guilt are likely to be actively fostered, whether directly (e.g. in the form of political vilification) or indirectly (e.g. in institutional forms of individualizing 'treatment').

It is often hard to see how these processes — of blame and guilt — operate within one's own experience. One tends to be caught up totally in blaming or feeling guilty, and it is frequently difficult to see how any other reaction could be more appropriate. Occasionally, however, perhaps even in the most trivial of situations, the blinkers slip a little, and one does indeed catch a glimpse of the wider view. I have not found it easy to think of examples, but perhaps the two following will do.

It has usually been part of my car-driving experience that in congested traffic conditions a certain, fairly high, percentage of drivers can be relied upon to make way for one to enter or leave a dense stream of traffic which otherwise, without their courtesy, would block one's progress for a long time. Usually, that is, someone will pause to make a gap for you to get into the stream or else to allow you to turn through or out of a stream in order, for instance, to enter a side-street. There is, however, one particular right turn I have to make on my way to work which involves turning across heavy traffic on the main road to enter a side road. The on-coming traffic through which I have to turn moves very slowly and haltingly, and all the car, bus and lorry drivers have a perfect view of my car patiently signalling its wish. It would cost none of these drivers any inconvenience or loss of time to pause to let me through, since they would be able immediately to catch up with the vehicles in front of them. And yet, absolutely consistently and day after day, they will crawl past nose-to-tail, stopping almost provocatively across the mouth of the side road, seeming nearly intentionally to block my getting into it. Drivers causing me this frustration will have been able easily to see for themselves that I have been waiting much longer than necessary to make this simple manoeuvre. Before I realized the inexorability of this phenomenon I used to fume with rage at the selfishness and lack of consideration of the on-coming drivers; every time someone eased to a halt across my bows I would mime sarcastic gratitude or perhaps even mouth a reproof. But it soon became clear that blame was not appropriate – it could not be the case that *all* these people were so brutally inconsiderate; there must be a *reason* for them to behave the way they did.

It was not until I happened to find myself in the same situation as the drivers who had so consistently frustrated me that I discovered what the reasons were. I found that their arrival at my usual turning-point is preceded by about half a mile of solid congestion, which may easily take fifteen to twenty minutes to negotiate. Though a car or two may be waiting to turn right across this agonizingly slow stream, their wait seems a relatively short one, and the roundabout ahead, which is the cause of the congestion, is tantalizingly close. When in *this* situation, the troubles of one or two would-be right turners seem as nothing when compared with *ours*!

We have, in other words, reasons for what we do, and they lie outside us. The 'selfishness' of a driver cannot be invoked as an explanatory concept out of the context of a situation in which he or she is to be found.

A woman I know whose job it is to be responsible for children in care, and who is as conscientious and concerned as anyone in this position could be, once described how she came to terms, in part at least, with her tendency to feel guilty over 'not caring enough' for her charges. She had had to go to a school open evening to discuss with the head teacher the almost total lack of progress of a twelve-year-old girl in her care. As she was waiting her turn she listened to a mother in front of her talking about the apparently very much more successful performance of her daughter. What struck my friend was the strength of this mother's *anxious concern*: clearly, she felt worried about her daughter in a way which was simply not possible for someone whose interest in a child was merely professional. She saw, in other words, that there were *reasons for* the relative indifference to 'her' children's school performance about which she had often felt guilty. Her guilt had consisted in a feeling that there was something lacking *inside her* which made it impossible to care properly for her charges, but as the result of this experience she was somewhat comforted by the realization that such feelings depend upon the *relation between* self and world. One cannot create in oneself certain forms of feeling just because they are thought desirable; the relation between mother and child is inescapably different from that between Child Care Officer and child, not only (and perhaps not most) because of the emotional bonds involved, but also because of the way being-a-parent is given shape by the social world in terms of the expectations, obligations, etc., it entails.

The structures of the world are experienced by us as *feelings*, and not as a series of intellectual, articulate appreciations. A parent *feels* the expectations and obligations of parenthood, and for most parents it would be both impossible and unnecessary for them to be able to 'unpack' these feelings into a verbal catalogue of their constituent parts. But we all, when placed in the appropriate situation, do experience the feelings, and because they are experienced personally, inside our own bodies, it is all too easy to form the mistaken impression that we as individuals are in some way totally responsible for them – i.e. that we are 'to blame' for them. To return for a moment to my example, because 'the system' renders her acquaintance with 'her' children inevitably intermittent and temporary, the Child Care Officer cannot be expected to feel caring about them in the same way as a parent whose connection with and commitment to her child is expected to be life long. The extent to which we 'care' is shaped by such issues as these, and not by some capacity within us for which we are somehow individually responsible. 'Caring' is not some kind of internal faculty, possession, emotional gift, or 'skill' – it is a complex phenomenon which stretches out beyond the individual who experiences it as a feeling into a network of external significations.

Over and over again we are seduced by the intimate internality of our experience into believing that the source of that experience is also to be found inside us, or that we can alter the nature of the experience by tinkering with our 'inner' workings. The fact that this is so easy to believe is quickly seized upon by the structures of interest as a way of mercilessly exploiting the world while leaving individuals preoccupied with personal guilt over the damage done: that huge proportion of humanity, for example, which must *inevitably* suffer privation if the powerful minority are to achieve 'happiness', may quite easily be led to feel that its miseries are caused not by the necessary consequences of social injustice, but by the personal failings of its members.

My unhappiness seems to stem from *inside* myself because that is where I *feel* it. Does it not therefore seem reasonable to suggest that it will best be alleviated through working on the internal feelings? This is a fundamental assumption of Western culture – and yet it is as sensible as looking for (and trying to change) the details of a picture in the camera that took it. We are so conditioned to accept this 'therapeutic assumption' (that unhappiness, or 'dysfunction', is to be 'cured' within the individuals who experience it) that to question it may earn one relegation to the lunatic fringe. Those who have, as for example Ivan Illich,* questioned the effectiveness as well as the rationality of a high technology medicine which attempts to 'cure' the world's ravages on our bodies merely by patching up the bodies themselves, have barely managed to obtain a hearing because it seems so 'obvious' that illness and disease are individual matters. (It is, at the same time, quite common for people to feel personal guilt or shame over being victims of disease.) Once again (and all the time) one must bear in mind that as well as being highly *plausible* (because of the way we experience our ills), the 'therapeutic assumption' is highly *convenient* because it allows us to plunder the world and exploit each other without having to be accountable for the damage we do in the process. Just as our 'memory of bliss' renders us vulnerable to the sales pitch of a society which depends for its continued viability on selling us 'happiness', so our bodily experience of pain and disease makes them only too intelligible as *individual* 'problems'; in both cases bodily experience combines with interest to mystify our understanding.†

*I. Illich, *Limits to Medicine*, Penguin Books, 1977.

†It is interesting in this respect to note the reception given by the British government to the report of the Working Party on Inequalities in Health set up, also by government, in 1977. The report shows that mortality rates for almost any category of disease or accident are much higher among the less advantaged members of society, and suggests that health inequalities on this scale cannot be explained 'except by invoking material deprivation as a key concept'. This of course implies that merely treating the damage after it has been done (the therapeutic assumption) fails to touch the root causes of ill health and injury, which are more accurately identified as consequences of socio-economic exploitation. The report has subsequently appeared in book form (P. Townsend and N. Davidson, eds., *Inequalities in Health*, Penguin Books, 1982), the editors noting that: 'The report was submitted to the Secretary of State in April 1980, but instead of being properly printed and published by the DHSS or HM Stationery Office, it was arranged for only 260 duplicated copies of the typescript to be publicly made available in the week of the August Bank Holiday in that year. Major organizations within the NHS, including health authorities, did not receive copies.' Such are the ways of repression!

In the case of psychological distress, the therapeutic assumption applies if anything even more powerfully than in the case of physical disease. This may in part be because *feelings* of distress or unhappiness are not seen as necessarily *bodily* things at all. Our mechanistic culture at least gives us a certain respect for the 'reality' of 'physical' entities like diseases, which we would on the whole not expect to be able to influence merely through the exercise of will or wishfulness, but when it comes to feelings, these seem to many so insubstantial as to be potentially much more amenable to quite easily conceived operations of will power or self control ('pull yourself together!'), or failing that, wise counsel and sympathetic therapy from the experts.

In fact, however, not only are we bodies, but we are bodies within a world. Our feelings, whether of joy or sorrow, ecstasy or pain, our most seemingly abstract intellectual and spiritual appreciations and accomplishments, our most finely tuned social sensibilities, all depend to be experienced at all on our bodily location within a particular spatio-temporal context (i.e. a situation and a history). I do not mean to say that our feelings are 'nothing but' physical events, that, for example, Beethoven's Fifth Symphony could in principle (or even best) be understood as a series of demonstrable events in his brain. This kind of crude mechanistic thinking has for too long obscured our understanding of the nature of human experience and achievement, and in fact relies on *dis*locating the human body from the world in which it is situated, precisely in order once again to emphasize individuality rather than relatedness. But it is equally absurd to disregard our embodiedness, to 'psychologize' our experience so that it becomes dislocated *and* disembodied – a play of imagery upon which, it seems, we can operate with the procedures of magic and fantasy to make of ourselves anything we wish.

We experience the world through our bodily engagement with it, and our conduct is for the most part the rational product of the physical structures of our bodies on the one hand and the social structures and exigencies of the world on the other. We can, it is true, *pretend* that the world is not as it is, and that our experience of it, especially when painful, is other than what we feel, and it may be (which was my theme in *Illusion and Reality*) that such pretence may become the norm, but in fact we cannot *escape* our suffering. However much we mystify our understanding and deceive ourselves about the meaning of our experience, there is in the last analysis absolutely no way in which we can avoid the consequences of being bodies within a world, and of knowing (even if we cannot say) what it is like to be such. It is this fundamental knowledge, the irreducible knowledge of the embodied subject, which affords us membership of a human community; however hard we may struggle to differentiate ourselves from our fellows, to render ourselves invulnerable to the terrible threats that human society creates, we can never really obliterate a knowledge of the truth of our situation, since it is given to us all in exactly the same way. However ingeniously we may play with words, seek to create objectivities on the one hand or relativities and perspectives on the other, we all know what it is like to feel cold, just as we bleed if you prick us. The 'truth', such as it is, of our situation lies, then, not in the discovery of some absolute reality beyond ourselves, nor in the constructions of our infinite ability to dream alternative worlds, but in the experience of the inescapable relation between our bodies and the context which envelops them.

Having for some years now watched, as attentively as I am able, people (including myself) struggling to feel and act differently from how they do feel and act, I am convinced that feeling and acting are far from being matters of will,* but are, as it were, held in place by the situation in which people find themselves – unless, that is, the person is in some way impelled to act contrary to reason. This is not to say that people's conduct is *determined* by their environment, but rather that they conduct themselves the way they do for good reasons. Determinism fails when applied to human conduct not so much because it is wrong as because it is logically inappropriate when applied to conscious beings: there is no conceivable situation in which human beings could have full knowledge of their circumstances and yet still be completely determined by them, and for this reason determinism becomes of no further relevance to psychology. On the other hand, this does not mean that we are free to do what we like or to feel what we want or think we ought to feel. We act and feel *rationally* according to our circumstances, and indeed our interests. To say that we act rationally is not to say that we act necessarily correctly or sensibly, but simply that we have reasons for what we do which follow from our experience of the world and our bodily relation to it.

The 'New Right' provides a good current example of the kind of moralism which makes use of the implausibility of mechanist determinism to instil in its victims a sense of guilt (self-blame) for their predicament, for it seems that if we are not *determined* by our environment to 'behave' the way we do, we must be *held responsible* for our 'freely' chosen responses to our world. But how 'free' people are to choose depends upon the range of choices open

*See in this respect L. H. Farber's wise little book, *Lying, Despair, Jealousy, Envy, Sex, Suicide, Drugs, and the Good Life*, Basic Books, 1976.

to them. My experience of people in psychological distress is that the combination of their history and their personal circumstances leaves them little reasonable alternative but to be distressed, just as if you let a naked man loose in the middle of the countryside in January he will be liable to feel cold, however 'free' he may in theory be to seek the equatorial sun or to imagine himself wrapped in a blanket before a blazing fire. In this way, the New Right uses banalized versions of eternal verities ('the freedom of the human spirit', etc.) to disguise a concerted and brutal attack precisely on what freedom people have by undermining the very grounds upon which they can rationally exercise it. To erode people's financial security, to limit their access to ideas and education, to impoverish their environments, swamp their consciousness with gutter propaganda and stupefy it with televisual soporifics, to constrain their protest through abuse of the law and its enforcement, and *then* to tell them to stand on their own two feet quite clearly constitutes cruel and cynical mystification. *Of course*, all things being equal, a person can be said to 'choose' those courses of action which he or she actually takes, but if the grounds upon which those choices are made are grossly skewed or distorted, he or she can scarcely be *blamed* for the direction taken. If apples cost five pence a pound and oranges five pounds, my choice of the former is neither forced by any mysterious process of determinism nor attributable to any particular moral quality I may possess – it is, even if highly predictable, merely rational.

Those people who, through their experience or expression of pain or confusion, fall into the arms of the 'helping professions', perhaps becoming psychiatrically diagnosed as psychotic or neurotic or 'inadequate personalities', have in my experience almost all arrived at their predicament through an entirely comprehensible, rational and (of course with hindsight) predictable process. If you run over a pea with a steam roller you don't blame the pea for what happens to it, nor, sensibly, do you treat its injuries as some kind of shortcoming inherent in its internal structure, whether inherited or acquired. Similarly, if you place the (literally) unimaginably sensitive organisms which human babies are in the kind of social and environmental machinery which we seem to be bent on 'perfecting', it can be of no real surprise that so many of them end up, as adults, as lost, bemused, miserable and crazy as they do. The only surprise, perhaps, is that so many pass as 'normal'.

The understanding which psychotherapists reach of the difficulties and unhappiness of their patients is unlikely to reveal any kind of absolute psychological 'laws', or any *necessarily* fundamental psychological 'problems'; what we find will depend as much upon the times we live in as upon any basic 'facts' about 'human nature'. It might well be, for example, that a psychological consultant to a closed and egalitarian order of peace-loving and scholarly monks would find himself focused upon issues of a quite different order from those facing the contemporary secular therapist – perhaps, for example, in that situation questions concerning the operation of the will would become paramount. In our situation, however, what can no longer be ignored, it seems to me, is the extent to which people are inevitably and in fact quite transparently damaged by the kinds of life which they cannot but be expected to 'choose' to lead. None of us, rationally, can escape the pursuit of happiness, nor the meshes of the net of interests through which we pursue it. What damages us are not our individual faults or shortcomings, but the instruments through which we wreak our inhumanity upon each other. We use our 'official' conceptualizations of the 'causes' of 'behaviour' to blind ourselves to – to repress – our involvement in a process of mutual exploitation and injury which serves the interests of a hierarchy of power.

In many respects the 'therapeutic assumption' constitutes an attempt to replace values of justice and equality (which make social demands upon us and place limits upon the extent to which we may indulge ourselves as individuals) with a reassurance that whatever harm the pursuit of happiness and self-interest may inflict can easily be put right. Furthermore, so deep within us is the therapeutic assumption established that even when a case for greater social justice and mutual care and compassion is conceded, we are still apt to say: 'That's all very well in the long term, but in the short term there are still all these inadequate and unhappy people who, damaged by the system though they may be, must still have something *done* about them.' In other words: 'Though therapy may not be the ultimate answer, we still need therapy.' We find it virtually impossible to *abandon* the idea of therapy, to contemplate *seriously* the possibility that in fact therapy may *really not work*. It is not just that such a possibility is seen as empirically unlikely: to voice it is liable to be taken by many as a kind of offence, if not against decency, then against fundamentally sane, rational discourse. And yet I think it may be true.

Even in my own reflections about patients I have known very intimately, I find it difficult to acknowledge that the circumstances which seem to attend real improvements in their 'condition' are the kind of thing which really *ought* to count as 'cure' – i.e. changes in the structure of their world such as job improvements, better housing, alterations in their personal relations (this, however, with provisos to be inferred from the discussion in Chapter 6). I still, in other words, find it hard to shake off a conviction that there ought to be some kind of 'pure' therapeutic change which stems directly and solely from the processes of therapy itself. I feel guilty that I cannot make magic.

But, like everyone else, my patients feel and act the way they do because they are bodies in a world, and only in so far as 'therapy' can affect *that* relation can it be of any help. On the whole, it is of much less help than almost any of us can bear to think. That is not necessarily quite such a bad thing as it sounds, for if therapy were as effective as we would like it to be – if the relation of the body with the world were so easily manipulated – human life would quickly be rendered almost entirely trivial. To gain a deeper understanding of these issues we need, I think, to examine the processes of 'change'.

5

Change: The Limits of Therapy

Psychotherapists have always had the greatest difficulty in demonstrating that their activities actually lead to anything remotely resembling a 'cure' of the 'conditions' presented by the patients who consult them. The focus of this book is not psychotherapy, and it is not my intention to try to deal exhaustively with the question of the usefulness or otherwise of the therapeutic enterprise as a whole; rather, I want to use the experience of therapy and therapists to examine the processes whereby people change. For nowhere do people try harder to change than in psychotherapy, and few people can have put more effort into trying to get other people to change than have psychotherapists.

There can, surely, be very few people who do not at some time in their lives want to change either the way they feel (because they feel distressed or unhappy) or the way they act (because alternative courses of action would be practically or morally preferable). But the possibility of change is not just important as a way of making life more pleasant, it seems also that flexible modification of characteristic forms of conduct will be necessary if people are to bring to bear an influence on the world. If we are to understand, and perhaps even give some deliberate direction to the way the social world evolves, we shall need to gain some kind of articulate idea of the ways in which people may change and how these may be facilitated. I do not believe that the kind of people who consult psychotherapists are particularly unusual, nor that the kinds of 'problems' they have are any different from anyone else's. Differences between the kinds of emotional pain and distress people feel, and whether or not they experience them through 'symptoms', are matters of degree rather than of kind. For these reasons, what one learns from the observation of people trying to change through psychotherapy almost certainly has, I believe, more general relevance. I suspect also that it is in the various ideas about change which psychotherapists have developed that the most 'sophisticated' psychological concepts concerning the processes of change in our culture are to be found. As will become apparent, this, I think, is not saying very much about the levels of sophistication psychologists have achieved in this respect.

There is a truly huge literature bearing upon research into the outcome of psychotherapy. For obvious reasons, it is very much in the interests of therapists to show that their procedures 'work', and most satisfactory of all would be if they could be shown to work straightforwardly as 'cures' in the way that we commonly conceive of cure in the field of physical medicine. However, as I have indicated, despite their best efforts psychologists and psychotherapists have been able to demonstrate no such simple achievement. Carrying out research in this field is by no means easy, and the complexities of research methodology are often cited as the main reason why results have not been encouraging, but few of those familiar with the literature could in good faith deny that therapeutic approaches have failed to live up to the hope once invested in them as 'cures'. Interestingly, this has not led to a lessening of therapeutic activity, nor, I think, to a lowering of expectations of therapy on the part of patients. Most therapists now agree that the 'does it work' question is far too oversimplified to allow of a sensible answer, and have become preoccupied instead with research into the *processes* of psychotherapy rather than its outcome, in the hope that a more intricate understanding of the kinds of events which take place in the 'therapeutic relationship' will lead to the formulation of more considered and sophisticated questions about change.

It is not my purpose here simply to attack or condemn psychotherapy as a means of offering help to people, but rather to indicate that the *kind* of help it offers cannot accurately be seen as one constituting a technology of change. I have no doubt at all that psychotherapy has a valid role to play within our society, but if we are to gain a clear idea of what is its value and what should be its place, and if, more importantly for present purposes, we are to understand better the processes whereby people actually do change, we need to absorb a little more honestly the lessons taught by the experience of psychotherapy, and question much more rigorously the grounds upon which we hold so tenaciously to the 'therapeutic assumption'. Most therapists, I suspect, have been rather traumatized by the research literature: the lack of hard evidence that any form of therapy really 'does any good' in the way that it is supposed to is something to set the seeds of panic sprouting in those who can see no obvious alternative way of making a living. Hence, the attempt by and large has been to explain this kind of evidence away rather than take it seriously and reflect on its significance. To do precisely this, however – to take it seriously – might lead to a considerable advance in our psychological understanding, and would not necessarily invalidate therapeutic activity itself, since therapy may have other uses than trying to change the way people are.

My own experience certainly accords with the findings of the research literature. What is striking, and at times even surprising, is precisely the extent to which patients do not change. This is not to say that people – whether 'patients' or not – do not change at all, but that, as I have already suggested, they do not change in the way and for the reasons that one might, on the basis of the best informed psychological 'knowledge', expect them to. This, I think, is because, in relation to change, the assumptions of both practical psychotherapy and the theoretical psychology it is based upon are almost entirely misleading, and entrenched in our thinking so deeply that we cannot make use of our actual experience of therapy in order to revise them. We insist that people must change in the ways we expect them to, rather than learning and intellectually elaborating the ways in which they actually do change. We are caught up in a psychological mythology which is designed to support our dreams of how we would like to be (and the structures of interest which maintain them) rather than developing a psychological science which takes serious account of what it finds. The practical upshot of our error is to persist in the construction of an ineffective and ultimately damaging psychological technology, rather than taking account in our moral conduct toward one another of the relative permanence of the damage we can inflict, and trying to avoid it.

There are, I think, three main strands to be identified in the accounts theorists of psychotherapy have put forward of the basic factors involved in change. These suggest that psychotherapeutic change may be brought about through the operation of (a) insight, (b) learning, and (c) love. The first two of these strands rest in essence on technological values, the third (far less widely represented) on a 'humanistic' view of the curative powers of relationship. In the actual practice (as opposed to the theoretical creed) of almost any kind of psychotherapy, one is likely to find all three of these strands at work, though in different proportions. The belief that they should 'work' in the sense of bringing about change owes much to the tradition of magic from which, as I suggested in Chapter 3, they may be traced.

The value of insight as a vehicle of change purely in itself is certainly less readily accepted by most thoughtful psychotherapists than it used to be, and yet many still work very hard to try to get their patients to achieve it, and I know from my own experience how difficult it is to overcome the frustration one feels when people at last come to see why they act and feel the way they do, and yet *still* persist in carrying on as before. There is a natural inclination, embedded as we are in a technological culture, for us to assume that we only need to know what the trouble is to be able to put it right – the greatest challenge appears to lie in the making of an accurate diagnosis. Patients, certainly, are frequently convinced that if only they can once discover what 'it' is which is troubling them it will be a simple matter to take the appropriate steps to recovery. Most of us in everyday life also probably subscribe to a tacit belief that a causal understanding of any particular emotional or 'relationship problem' leads more or less automatically to a prescription for effective adjustment.

Some of the early literature on psychoanalysis testifies to an enthusiastic confidence in the power of insight simply to evaporate so-called neurotic 'symptoms' – once the patient accepted that, say, her functional paralysis was related to an infantile wish to sleep with her father, it would simply disappear. Whether or not such spectacular cures were then achieved, they are certainly hard to come by now, and most therapists today recognize that knowledge of the history of a 'problem' is not of itself sufficient to make it go away. Hence the importance of learning. Even if you know very well why you act and react in the way that you do, you still, in order to change, have to *learn* to act differently.

I have no doubt that learning is indeed the single most fundamentally important factor in the kind of self-initiated change which psychotherapy seeks to achieve, and yet, because of their need to justify their activity in terms of a *technical* rhetoric (which in turn contains a still compelling appeal to magic) therapists have handled the concept of learning very badly. For the most part, they have cast the processes of learning in almost entirely mechanistic categories, and have thus reinterpreted them in terms of training or conditioning. In this way, it is expected that 'faulty responses' may, through an appropriate course of training designed, naturally, by therapists who are experts in the relevant 'laws', be replaced by more 'adaptive' ones. There are many varieties of mechanist vocabulary in which this fundamental idea is expressed, and it would be unnecessarily tedious for me to attempt to outline them here, but they all add up to more or less the same thing. At the present time, the most widespread version of human beings as 'learning machines', and one which has penetrated deep into popular culture, is that which characterizes people as bundles of 'skills' whose acquisition is, for the most part, a matter of obtaining the necessary training from the appropriate experts.

Virtually any competence or ability which can be named, including those which involve our dealings with others, comes to be broken down into some more or less plausible combination of 'skills'. Thus we have 'interpersonal skills' and 'social skills' along with 'language skills' and 'footballing skills'. There is, of course, something immensely reassuring about a 'skills' model of human activity: for those needing to acquire some, it becomes merely a matter of getting the right input from a relevant training source, and for those whose job it is to purvey knowledge the whole matter of teaching and learning becomes a relatively simple one of 'skills transmission'. In this way training, or learning, becomes conceived of as in principle no more complicated than popping a program into a computer. Programs may be popped in or out, erased or replaced, according to whatever skills you or your trainers may consider it desirable for you to have at any particular time.

Despite the fact that there is a very deliberate and extremely heavy investment within 'official' psychology in the people-as-computers model of psychological functioning, it seems to me that the propensity of ordinary people to consider themselves as programmable vehicles of skills has developed alongside rather than as the result of any campaign on the experts' part to popularize such a view. Quite why this should be so is unclear, but it is striking how readily, and with what an unself-consciously smug satisfaction, people talk about the skills they 'have' or intend to 'polish up', etc. Suddenly, and quite without noticing it, we appear to have entered a world in which people can talk without absurdity of, for instance, going on a course to 'acquire management skills', and having been on it, can in all seriousness and in the correct anticipation of being 'credible', list their mere attendance at the course on their CVs as *evidence* of their acquisition of the skills in question. There is here, it seems, an interlocking of the interests of trainers and learners, in a society where there is in fact not enough of importance to train or learn, such that both subscribe, symbiotically as it were, to an illusion. In an economy which depends upon the highly artificial production and consumption of worthless tokens of 'happiness' (and in particular upon the 'management' of such production and consumption), it is precisely because there is to be found no real appreciation of skill at anything that we are able to convince each other that we are the proud possessors of such a variety of 'skills'. Because our society has drifted so far from preserving and encouraging in its members activities of any real meaning or value, we collude in a kind of collective fantasy of achievement and ability.

In psychotherapy likewise, though not perhaps always quite so crassly, the assumption is that 'learning to be different', though not necessarily easy, involves an erasure or replacement of experience, as though, again, experience were acquired in the manner of tape recording. In this way, therapists, and indeed their patients, may expect that through facing up to 'problems' or practising new 'responses' to old 'stimuli', patients' 'maladaptive behaviour' and the experience which maintained it will be wiped out. This mechanistic approach to learning, though certainly it is not without some therapeutic value, is much too simplistic, and in my view grossly underestimates the enormous *difficulty* of change. The difficulty is, of course, that we are not computers, and our conduct is not the result of any kind of erasable programming. This is a point to which I shall return shortly.

Implicit in some currently quite influential varieties of psychotherapy (so-called 'cognitive' therapies) is a kind of combination of 'insight' and 'learning' assumptions which results in the view that psychological or emotional distress is best dealt with by learning to take an alternative view of things. This really amounts to nothing more than a variant on the maxim 'look on the bright side', and since I have dealt with its inadequacies at some length in *Illusion and Reality* I shall not go into greater detail now. Here again, however, what seems to be suggested is that people's distress is generated from a program somehow buried inside their heads, that what matters is the way they see things rather than the way things are.

The failure of attempts based on the operation of insight and learning to change 'behaviour' and alleviate distress in any consistently demonstrable way, despite the often plausible claims made and the plethora of techniques spawned by the various therapeutic schools, has led some therapists to pass beyond a purely technical view of change to consider the significance of the personal relationship between patient and therapist.

There is little doubt, I think, that the personal influence of therapist on patient, and indeed of patient on therapist, is a highly potent factor in nearly all forms of psychotherapy, whether theoretically acknowledged or not. There could be no more superfluous statement of the obvious than that, in all kinds of relationship and in all kinds of spheres, people are profoundly affected by other people. Psychotherapy is no exception, and there has always been a significant minority of psychotherapists who have insisted on making the personal relationship between therapist and patient central to an understanding of therapeutic help.* There can be very few psychotherapists who have failed to notice the importance patients attach to their opinion of them and the extent to which people may blossom under and draw courage from the 'positive regard', as Carl Rogers called it, of the therapist. Even Freud (who is not usually credited with obvious 'humanistic' tendencies), in his

---

*Valuable accounts of this kind have more recently been given by Peter Lomas, *The Case for a Personal Psychotherapy*, Oxford University Press, 1981, and R. F. Hobson, *Forms of Feeling. The Heart of Psychotherapy*, Tavistock Publications, 1985. See also my *Psychotherapy: A Personal Approach.*

study of the 'rat man' betrays an awareness of the effect on his patient of an expression of warmth: 'In this connection I said a word or two upon the good opinion I had formed of him, and this gave him visible pleasure'.*

Some writers on psychotherapy† have overcome professional reticence sufficiently to be able to suggest that it is essentially the power of love that lies behind therapeutic potency, but while I would certainly not want to quarrel with the view that patients are indeed moved by therapists' affection and concern, and that their self-confidence may be greatly boosted and their resolve to tackle their difficulties strengthened, the degree to which ultimately they do move is still often disappointing. I must say again that I do not by this mean to belittle the value of therapeutic love, but only to suggest what should be the limits of the claim it makes. I have no wish to deny that in some sense or other – perhaps in many senses – psychotherapy may be 'good for' people, but I do wish to question how far it *changes* them, and further, I wish strongly to cast doubt on any assumption that it 'cures' them.

It is a very frequent experience that patients who have felt quite seriously disturbed for months or even years may feel an enormous sense of relief and improvement following their first consultation with a sensitive and attentive psychotherapist. For a few days their troubles seem to fall away as if by magic. But this state, sadly, does not last for long: the initial relief at finding a sympathetic ear, the surge of joy at feeling less alone, quickly recede as the world closes in again and the features of it which were causing the distress in the first place reassert their claims. Of course, in one's battles with the world, it helps to find an intelligent, experienced, wise and loving ally, and those adequately provided with such (especially early in their lives) will never need a psychotherapist. But allies of this calibre are, in the present-day world, in desperately short supply, and if you need one badly enough the chances are you will have to pay for one.

For all the technical mystique psychotherapists have managed to erect around themselves, for all the reverential awe in which they have, sometimes rather sentimentally, managed to intone their rhetoric of love, for all, even, the draining and dedicated effort they put into what is often a very demanding job, they are still but weakly allies. Unlike (in ideal circumstances) family or friends, therapists play an only temporary role in the lives of almost all their patients, and their commitment to help is strictly limited in

---

*S. Freud, Notes upon a case of obsessional neurosis. Pelican Freud Library, vol. 9.

†See for example I. D. Suttie, op. cit.

terms of their actual involvement in patients' lives (were this not so, the job would become demanding beyond endurance). To talk of love in these circumstances is to edge close to hypocrisy, and indeed I strongly suspect that the efficacy of therapeutic love is strictly proportional to the real commitment of therapists to their patients. Though in almost all ways the comparison is far from fair, it is nevertheless not totally irrelevant in this respect to point to the worlds of difference there are between Mother Teresa of Calcutta and the average Hampstead psychoanalyst (and the supposed technical expertise of the latter in no way matches in therapeutic potency the commitment of the former).

Therapeutic love may, I think, most accurately be seen as a convenient, and infinitely less effective, substitute for the real thing. Therapists are liable quite happily to talk of 'corrective emotional relationships', of patients reliving, and somehow exorcizing the traumata of their infancy under their therapists' soothing tutelage, and though such talk is, I am sure, uttered with complete sincerity and in the best of faith, I think the time has come for us to acknowledge that there is really not a shred of convincing evidence to support it, and nor would one expect there to be.

On the question of 'cure', not all psychotherapists are as confident as I may have seemed to suggest. Roy Schafer, for instance, comes very close to the position I am adopting here:

> . . . while the past may be partially re-experienced, reviewed, and altered through reinterpretation, it cannot be replaced: a truly cold mother, a savage or seductive father, a dead sibling, the consequences of a predominant repressed fantasy, years of stunted growth and emotional withdrawal, and so forth, cannot be wiped out by analysis, even though their hampering and painful effects may be greatly mitigated, and the analysand freed to make another, partly different and more successful try at adaptation. The analysand whose analysis has been benignly influential retains apprehensions, vulnerability, and characteristic inclinations toward certain infantile, self-crippling solutions, however reduced these may be in influence and however counterbalanced by strengthened adaptiveness.*

But nestling innocently even in this far from over-optimistic text is the view that patients may be 'freed' from a past which is (magically) alterable through reinterpretation, and once again we see the therapeutic assumption refusing in the end to relax its grip.

For while therapy may be or achieve all kinds of things – it may

---

A New Language for Psychoanalysis, op. cit.

be comforting, encouraging, inspiring, healing of hurt – one thing it cannot do is free people from their past, because people are not computers with programs which can simply be removed and replaced.

Not only are people extremely resistant to the kind of change which we see as the hoped-for result of therapeutic 'adaptation', but it is highly undesirable that they should be anything else. Only if one unquestioningly accepts an individualistic view that all that matters is the personal happiness people manage to achieve in a particular lifetime can one feel anything but nervous about the prospect of a really effective technology of change. It is, after all, far from obvious that we yet know what form of society is truly good for us, and if there is to be a sufficient range of conduct and experience within humanity to ensure a future which makes possible the evolution of a *variety* of (at present unknowable) social developments, it is important that *particular* lines of experience and conduct are pursued doggedly, not only throughout individuals' lives, but from one generation to the next. If we really were as easily alterable as many therapeutic systems (as well as other more sinister techniques of change) would have us believe, there can be little doubt that a politically dominant power group would quickly establish those norms of 'personality' and 'behaviour' which best served its interests.

This, of course, is exactly what politically dominant power groups already try to do (and not without a degree of success) but they do it by standardizing the environment, not people. In this respect, the modern state which attempts to control people through a standardization of their environment, shows a more sophisticated understanding of 'what makes people tick' than do professional therapists who focus their attentions on what is inside people's heads. In this way, a standardized, uniform 'psychology' is likely to be established much more easily by controlling what goes into people's heads than by trying to alter it once it has got there. Television is a much more powerful means of ensuring uniformity of belief than was the Inquisition, and the mentality which invented factory farming is not slow to appreciate the regularity and predictability to be achieved by standardizing experiential as well as nutritional diet. Used to it though one is, it is still quite an eerie experience to walk round any residential suburb after dark and to note the extent to which people are imbibing exactly the same impressions and information from the glowing screens; one only has to check the evening's programme to know what people will be talking about the next morning.

To try to alter people's experience after they have acquired it is a bit like trying to control the weight of battery chickens by surgery

– in fact the latter would be by far the easier task. The fact is that people are organisms and their experience is acquired organically, and so deeply and inextricably bound up is it with the very structures of the body that erasure of the experience would entail destruction of the organism. We cannot, like magnetic tape, be wiped clean of our history, which is, on the contrary, acquired as are the growth rings of a tree. Our history, the knowledge we have built up of the world, *is* our physical, organic structure. Body and mind are not just inseparable, they are one and the same.

It is certainly an expectation of our therapeutic culture that somehow our painful experience can be eradicated, or at least that the misery we feel in the present can somehow be wiped away to leave us with a 'clean slate' on which to start to chalk up a new and more promising future. Only an entirely unreflective ideology of mechanism allows us to think in this way and to shut our eyes to the obvious fact that our present feelings and perceptions have a history which is, as it were, deeply and ineradicably inscribed upon our bodies. In clinging on to a therapeutic illusion, we exempt those aspects of our conduct and experience we would like magically to change from rules of common sense which we would think it close to madness not to apply in other, related areas. Our ability to construct a social world at all depends on our being able correctly to anticipate a high degree of regularity and predictability in the character and conduct of other people. It is in many ways important that leopards should not be able to change their spots, and it is certainly our experience that they do not. Nor do any of us expect to be able to change as the result of any kind of 'therapeutic' intervention the way we speak, or move, or argue, think, interpret, react, and we pursue our aims, enact our abilities and competences, speak languages and ride bicycles without expecting ever to be 'cured' of doing so. It is not, of course, that there is no possibility of our being able to learn new and different ways of doing things, but in learning of this kind we anticipate the *difficulty* involved in a way which is less characteristic of our therapeutic aspirations, and we also know that what we learn does not expunge (again, in the manner of magnetic tape) what was there before.

Over and over again the rooted, organic nature of our experience has been misinterpreted as indicative of some form of malfunction or maladjustment. If people do not operate in a *mechanically* adaptable way in relation to some particular set of circumstances defined (usually by a professional group) as ideal, they are seen as somehow resistant or faulty, for example as demonstrating 'transference neurosis', 'inappropriate conditioning', etc. However, a person is not formed by what goes on physically or psychologically inside his or her own skin, but from a highly permeable relation with a context – the world in which we are situated flows into us and we into it in a way which makes us inseparable from it, and which is indelibly recorded in our history. This is the basis of the importance to human beings of familiarity; we make sense of and struggle with and grow from our roots in whatever world we happen to be, and to have been, located. You will not want to exchange your Belfast back street for a desert island paradise not because you are crazy or stupid, but because your experience is inseparable from the one and irrelevant to the other. We can only deal with what we know. If you suspect that all men are bullying tyrants as your father was, this is not so much a mistake you are making as a particular, and quite valid, form of knowledge you are not merely unwilling, but, as it were, organically unable to abandon. Our bodies make sure that we do not forget the lessons of our past. I do not want to say that people are incapable of developing or modifying experience as they go through life, but that such development or modification must fit in with and grow out of what has gone before – it must be organic. People *grow* from one position to the next, they cannot be *switched*. Our experience is hard won, built into our living tissue, and it should be respected rather than measured disparagingly against a set of professional norms of 'adjustment' or 'mental health'.

Unhappily for those who place their hopes in therapy, the lessons of our exposure to pain, deprivation, injustice and misfortune, are registered as indelibly on our bodies as are those of love, security and nurturance, and indeed as are those practical acquisitions (like learning a mother tongue or being able to swim) which we tend to take for granted. There is no difference in terms of the quality of the knowledge itself between what an insecure and anxious person *knows* about the world in terms of its brutality and unpredictability, and what a secure and confident person *knows* about its potentialities for affection and achievement. There is no reason at all why one should consider the one person's experience and expectations 'pathological' and the other's 'adjusted', except of course that a confusion of social with *quasi* medical values makes it much easier to ignore the harm we do each other and to establish a uniform view that any casualties which may occur in what purports to be a fundamentally benign society are solely the result of individual 'dysfunction', inappropriate 'projection', and so on.

It is, of course, against the interests of a hierarchy of power which depends on exploitation for people to recognize that the distress or despair they feel stems from their bodily relatedness to a noxious world, since any such recognition, should it occur on a wide enough scale, would quickly lead to demands for social change. In view of this one must note again that, paradoxically, the fact that people are so resistant to therapeutic change has a positive value: even if a kind of uniformity and docility can be imposed through the unification of experience (as through television) the actual suffering caused by the injustices and inequalities of our society cannot easily be concealed under a blanket of therapy. People cannot but register what happens to them, and they cannot but spend their lives following out its significance. In some respects, then, we are less easily turned into battery chickens than one might fear. I do not, of course, wish to suggest that suffering is a good thing, only that perhaps it is good that mystification of the reasons for it may still meet with considerable resistance.

However, though therapy does not 'work' in the way that we would like it to, it is still difficult to cast doubt upon its efficacy without appearing to be cruel. To say that a person's distress arises, at least in so far as it is historically rooted, out of ineradicable experience seems to be close to condemning him or her to a lifetime of unhappiness; after all, our society runs on the expectation that, in principle at least, happiness is attainable for all. In fact, however, it is my experience that more often than not people meet the 'truth' of their predicament with relief, and that what is most painful to deal with is not the difficulty – even tragedy – of our situation, but the tantalizing but empty promise of its betterment or 'cure'. I have often been, and I am sure shall continue to be, amazed at the fortitude and resilience of people who discover that what they thought was a curable illness is in fact the outcome of an unalterable history and (usually) a highly inimical set of circumstances which may be desperately hard if not impossible to influence. Most people are *glad* to be rid of the mystification which prevented them from understanding and getting to grips with, often, appallingly difficult features of their past and present, and enormously relieved if they find someone who will share with them an unflinching view of cruelties and injustices whose marks they will always bear.

The errors of our mechanized and wishful view of ourselves are very often more damaging than the injuries they are designed to conceal. It is on the face of it paradoxical that a culture which so much stresses individuality for the purposes of promoting 'happiness' and instilling blame, should at the same time, through the imposition of uniformity and the standardization of 'normality', make it so difficult for people to accept and allow for the uniqueness of their experience. For example, because, in a standardized society, we not unreasonably take our own experience as the standard for all, we tend to have a tacit expectation that we should be instantly 'understandable' by others. If, then, you do not 'understand' me, it must be because of some unusual obtuseness or quirk of personality on your part. We have very little tolerance for the differences there are between us, the differences which, presumably, stem from the organic relation of each of us with varying sets of circumstances. Many people, indeed, live their lives in a kind of perpetually terrified comparison with a non-existent norm. Thus people may spend a lifetime trying to achieve an objective standard (as human being) which in fact does not exist at all, and in so doing by-pass, discount or try to invalidate their own subjective experience. But subjective experience is inescapably rendered by one's embodiment in a world, and the attempt to replace it with some form of normative, 'objective' ideal is likely to result in either a kind of mad artificiality or else torments of confusion and despair.

If therapy cannot cure our distress it can, in some cases at least, clear our confusion, and once this has been achieved it may be possible for some people to engage with the world, or to change their situation within it, in a way which leads to its impinging upon them less painfully. For a small proportion of articulate and socio-economically advantaged people, it may even be that psychotherapy has value as an insight-giving procedure enabling them to see and act upon idiosyncrasies of their history or mistakes of interpretation about the significance of factors in their past or present circumstances. But therapeutic benefit of this kind arises only because such people have *available to* them (not *inside* them) the freedom to do something about their lives. If this is so it is, I think, of very little general relevance, if only because people in difficulties of this kind are very likely eventually to work them out and put them right for themselves.

For the vast majority of people who are driven to despair (whether they know it or not) by the nature of our society, the means of rectification of their predicament are usually beyond their own resources. One should not because of this underestimate the value psychotherapy might have as a means of clarifying their situation and offering comfort in their contemplation of it, but nor should one overestimate its ability to change them. As far as change is possible, it is likely to be achieved only with great difficulty. We have been misled by our metaphor of mechanical change to ignore almost totally the difficulties inherent in organic change and to overlook the extent to which its possibilities are limited by both the environment and the bodily history in which we are organically rooted. Perhaps we can, with painful effort, learn to do differently some things which we learned to do unproductively or self-destructively, but we would be foolish to overlook the influence of the world around us.

We would do better to see ourselves as plants rather than as machines, and we might benefit from applying to our own lives some very elementary rules of horticulture. Any kind of treatment for plants which consisted solely of attempting alterations to their internal structure would be unlikely to recommend itself to gardeners. Plants grow best in well understood and carefully prepared conditions – of sun or shade, damp or dryness, heat or cold, in this or that kind of soil. A plant which grows poorly or mis-shapenly may well be improved through careful attention to its environment, provision of light or water, but it will still bear the scars of an inauspicious beginning. I do not want to overwork the analogy, but it does seem strange to me that we should often lavish so much more attention on our gardens than on our fellow beings and our progeny. Nobody expects their cauliflowers to grow by magic.

The alternative to reliance on a technology of change is the cultivation of a society which takes care of its members. If we cannot cure the damage we have done we can try to mitigate its effects on future generations, and to achieve this we have to recognize the importance of the conditions in which we live and the way we conduct ourselves towards each other.

6

'Relationships'

By far the greater part of the misery which is experienced by people in the modern world is unquestionably inflicted through human agency. It is the things we do to each other which are the immediate causes of our distress. Superficially, therefore, it might seem as though one need look no further than our 'relationships' one with another to identify, and in principle also to rectify, the origins of our unhappiness.

At no time in previous history, certainly, have 'relationships' so directly been a focus of concern and discussion as in our own time. Entire industries have grown up around our ability, or lack of ability, to attract or be pleasing to others and to enjoy what they have to offer us. Not the least important section of this market is that exploited by the therapy industry: 'interpersonal relationships' are acknowledged as the core concern of a hundred different 'schools' of therapy and counselling, and not surprisingly so, for anxious rumination about one's personal adequacy in relation to others, dread of rejection by them and frustration at lack of satisfaction in 'relationships' seem to lie at the very centre of much of our acute personal unhappiness. For most of us our 'relationships' – or at least our fantasies of how they might or ought to be – seem to constitute the very meaning of our existence: life would appear to have no point at all were it not for the promise it holds of satisfying personal relationships.

However, far from exposing or providing an understanding of the nature of our predicament, this pervasive, almost obsessive concern with 'relationships' seems to me actually itself to form a large part of what ails us. Indeed, our desperation to enjoy 'good relationships' lies behind a great deal of the damage we do each other, and constitutes much more a reflection than a critique of social values stemming from the commercialized pursuit of happiness.

The commercial process turns abstractions like 'happiness' into saleable commodities. In exactly this way, abstract relations between people have been turned into 'relationships' which are treated as the end-product of a process in which people themselves form the raw material. Thus people have become secondary to the relationships of which, interchangeably and expendably, they form a part: what matters is the 'quality of the relationship', not the characteristics or conduct, or even ultimately the welfare, of the people who form its terms.

The language we use testifies to this state of affairs quite clearly. 'My relationship is breaking up'; 'I think she's looking for a new relationship'; 'they've got a really good relationship'. The following extract from an advertisement for one company's 'double cassette twin-pack courses' puts the issue at its most vulgarly basic:

MAKE AN IMPRESSION!

This course deals with all aspects of self-presentation, whether in the workplace or in social or family life. The idea of 'self-marketing' is a major theme and situations in which the skills have an important role include:

Y   starting and maintaining relationships

Y   interview training

Y   self-presentation in groups

Y   developing closer relationships

Y   building better interactions at work

Y   handling rejection effectively

Y   establishing arenas for 'self-marketing'

Y   making and clarifying agreements with others.

This, then, is the 'arena' where people ('selves') have become caught up in a commercialized and competitive jockeying for position, in which the adequacy of 'self-presentation' will determine how satisfactory 'relationships' are, and in which the terrors of rejection may be 'handled effectively' through development of the appropriate 'skills'.

As the virtually inexhaustible supply of raw material for saleable satisfactions in the form of 'relationships', people become almost less than commodities, and this no doubt accounts for the intense and obsessive anxiety which they experience over their relations with others. Usually from bitter experience, most people know how easily dispensed with they are as those 'significant others' with whom they come into contact during their lives seek *through* them the satisfaction of their needs. At the centre of our anxiety, then, is to be found the terror that we shall simply *disappear* if we are not wanted, needed, or 'loved' by someone. Our very sense of identity and existence depends upon the gaze of someone else falling upon us – and it is noticeably with identity and existence that twentieth-century people, as well as much of their literature, art, psychology and philosophy, have been particularly preoccupied. We are objects, and as such have to be *noticed* in order to achieve full 'objectivity'. Objects exist only for others; only subjects can exist independently of the regard of 'the Other'. And, of course, we use others in precisely the way we fear they may use us – we treat them not as ends in themselves, but as means to more or less satisfactory 'relationships'. As far as you do not satisfy some aspect of my needs, you do not exist for me. In other words, if one is nobody's object one is, quite literally, nothing. The value of people thus becomes entirely utilitarian – if they are no use to anyone, they are simply expendable. It is no longer human lives which are important, but the quality of the relationships and satisfactions to which they contribute.

Our acceptance of the expendability of people who fail to contribute to our personal happiness is perfectly obvious if one examines the content of our fantasy. In the media of popular entertainment, for example 'successful' television drama, characters are kept in existence only so long as they contribute to the sexual or material satisfaction of the protagonists. In the glossier American television series, moreover, these vehicles of gratification are completely interchangeable, conforming to a standard mould of youth and 'beauty' which, even though it makes them hard to tell apart, becomes the heartbreakingly unattainable ideal of those more normally fashioned viewers who dread being exposed as substandard. And one should not be led by the tastelessness of such fantasies as these into believing that they bear no relation to the values we really hold dear – indeed, their very popularity betrays the coarse directness of their celebration of what we have come to be interested in.

Up until very recently there seemed to be little conscious aware-ness among people I saw as patients (whom, again, I single out only because I know them best, not because I see them as different from the rest of us) that the injuries they occasioned and incurred in the course of their pursuit of happiness were anything other than the necessary result of failures in 'relationship'. People longed for relationships they fancied they had never had, or pined for lost relationships they feared they would never have again. They fretted and seethed over frustrating relationships they could no longer abide, they struggled with the panicky loss of identity consequent on scarcely having any relationships at all, or they tried desperately to piece themselves together after emerging from years of being the victim of punitive or destructive relationships. In nearly all cases these seemed to be 'relationship problems' arising more or less directly out of human nature itself, and the 'answer' to them seemed to lie in 'finding a good (or better) relationship'. All that was needed, so it seemed, was love.

Now there are, I think, signs of a change taking place: no longer do patients see 'the problem' quite so much as one of being on the wrong side of a split between 'good' and 'bad' relationships, but rather they begin to articulate a sense that there is something not right with the very concept of relationship itself. This feeling tends to be expressed in one of two ways: either in complaints that our relations with each other are *generally* bad and that the world has become a place of brutality and indifference from which there appears to be no haven, or in a conviction that the game of 'relating' has become no longer worth the candle, that *any* kind of relationship, good, bad or indifferent, somehow imposes an intolerable strain. I sometimes get the feeling that where not long ago people longed to be loved, they now long to be left in peace.

Whether or not this is so, and I certainly do not wish to make a major issue of it, it would not be a particularly surprising or unpredictable result of our 'commodification' of relationships, for anything one tries in this way to elevate into being the point of our lives is bound in the end to turn to dust and ashes. Just as one is bound to generate despair by trying to turn the 'epiphenomenon' of happiness into a concretely attainable commodity, so attempting to make abstract relations between people into 'marketable' sources of satisfaction is certain in the end to lead to a situation in which people are in fact treated with heartless unconcern or are experienced as objects of frustration.

Our mistake has been not to see – or to forget – that relations become established between people not as ends in themselves but in the course of doing something else. Over and over again we try to turn actions into entities, conduct into commodity, abstract into concrete, quality into quantity. This, of course, not out of wilfulness or stupidity, but because we are immersed in a society which depends for its continued functioning on the manufacture of satisfactions and the manipulation of interests. The state of the consumer's nervous system becomes the most potent 'variable' in the selling process: if there are pleasant sensations attached to any form of activity, including activities which we pursue together (i.e. relatedly), they must be isolated, commodified and brought into the market-place. We no longer see people as there to do things with or for, but as the interchangeable terms of relationships which may be more or less satisfying. Love itself ceases to have a *function* in the moral sphere of human conduct but becomes a kind of gratification of need to be sought or even extorted from people as a good rather than striven after as a form of commitment *for the sake of* something beyond personal satisfaction.

The fate of our 'relationships' provides another example of what happens when human beings are deprived of a function in the world – when, that is, the possibilities open to people to act on their environment are, so to speak, drained out of their embodied existence and re-presented to them as mechanized commodities for their consumption. Those things which we could do together are done for us and sold back to us in the form of entertainment, spectacle or consumer goods. Our communal activities, those things which we could do in relation with each other, thus become empty, collapsed in on themselves, literally without meaning. Our relatedness is overcome by a kind of paralysing self-consciousness because it can no longer point beyond itself to any kind of purpose.

The most satisfying relationships are again probably those of which the participants are almost entirely unaware. Even though opportunities for activity giving rise to relationship of this kind have become pitifully rare, most of us have probably had the experience of doing things with someone – working, perhaps, or playing – in which the complementary abilities and contributions of the participants achieved a result which neither could possibly have managed alone, and which led, almost certainly retrospectively, to an awareness of warmth and appreciation which never needed to be mentioned. It would seem completely artificial for friends, or lovers, or spouses, suddenly to stop dead in the course of their mutual activity to comment on the quality of their relationship, and yet, more and more, this is exactly what is happening. Partly because there seems to be so little of value *to* do and partly because we have become objects of gratification for each other, we spend more and more time talking and thinking about our 'relationships' rather than doing anything with them. It may help in thinking about this state of affairs to consider one at a time some of those spheres of relationship which have been rendered particularly problematic by our social organization.

Friendship

With one or two notable exceptions – for example the American psychiatrist H. S. Sullivan – friendship is a form of relationship little discussed in the 'clinical literature' of psychology and psychiatry, though loneliness and isolation play a very prominent role in the kinds of emotional distress which drive people to seek help from the 'experts'. The ideal 'therapeutic' solution to such loneliness is often seen as the formation of a long-term sexual bond, and when most people talk of their need to establish 'a relationship' what they usually mean is an exclusive liaison with someone of the opposite sex. In this way, and with consequences I shall come to consider shortly, heterosexual pair-relationships carry a very heavy *therapeutic* load in our society: warmth, safety, fulfilment and

97

'understanding' are the hoped-for results of shutting yourself cosily away with your lover.

Outside this kind of exclusive, sexually based therapeutic intimacy (as it turns out, itself largely fantasy) the development of friendly relations with others appears to be problematic, particularly in the adult population. The reason for this, it seems to me, again cannot be put down to the internal characteristics of individuals, but to a social organization which renders adult life, for most people, both competitive and aimless. We compete in 'the market' for satisfactions and empty tokens of achievement which in practice dictate that our activity has no aim beyond its own temporary satiation. It is thus impossible for the vast majority of people to find anything to do together in which they can collaborate wholeheartedly, unreflectively and constructively. Those activities around which friendships may be formed tend of necessity to be contrived leisure-time pursuits, failing which friendships must be manufactured self-consciously as ends in themselves. Apart from this, relations between people are characterized by a kind of watchful hostility as they compete with each other in the struggle to gain recognition of an artificially constructed pseudo-identity. In a world organized exclusively around commercial and material interests, the focus of concern for the individual becomes the *self* and the gratification which may follow from ministration to its appearance ('presentation of self') and its needs (the ideal of the quiescent nervous system). It is only when people are able to focus beyond themselves as objects on to a goal or aim in pursuance of which they may *lose* themselves, that they may join in collaborative, as opposed to competitive, activity with others. It is probably for this reason that the most rewarding friendships made tend to be at times of one's life, for example childhood, adolescence or (particularly perhaps for some women) young parenthood, when one finds oneself thrown together with other people in activity which is at least not completely dominated by the ethics of the market-place.

I wonder if men have particular difficulty in making friends. My experience with male patients leads me to suspect that the much-maligned characteristics of masculine insensitivity and emotional unresponsiveness are much more the consequence of spiritually mutilating economic values than of any inherently macho personality features of men themselves, or indeed of any real advantage in power or status to be gained by toughness. In fact we have all – men and women – been driven by ruthless economic competition, and by the unavoidable demands which have been placed upon us to cherish our selves, to retreat into the last embattled refuge of tenderness, i.e. sex, where undefended intimacies may, if but briefly, be exchanged. In other times and places men seem to have been no more reticent than women in expressing their (non-sexual) love for others, and my patients (and indeed nearly all the men I have got to know intimately) experience the necessity to be stereotypically male as an imposition rather than an advantage. But the hierarchy of power is held in place by occult violence, not by love, and its values must be reproduced in the individuals who are shaped to maintain it; men are its victims no less than women.

Because there is relatively so little scope for the unself-conscious generation of friendship through cooperative absorption in constructive activity, our need for friendship has often to be met artificially. For friendship, which might once have been a, so to speak, inevitable accident of social relations, an unreflected-upon bonus of communal life, has now indeed become a *need*. If the point of life is the celebration of self, one cannot do without others with whom to celebrate; if others are not there to confirm my identity, to reflect my image, I just disappear. As friends we are, then, mirrors to each other, taking turns to reflect our images back at each other, entering, for the sake of our emotional survival, a kind of cowardly pact not to break the rules by saying what we really see. Like schoolboys in a boxing match who secretly agree not to hurt each other, we nervously acquiesce in a mutual lowering of defences on condition only that we shall not criticize. This kind of fake mutuality is quite explicitly advocated in some half-baked North American forms of 'therapy', and results in some quite extraordinarily false types of 'relationship' in which the hollow exchange of reciprocal 'strokes' is quite likely to end in a burst of bitter recrimination when one of the participants can no longer stand the dishonesty and begins to tell the truth.

Increasingly, the precarious fragility of our 'self-images' and the pervasive treachery of our competitive social existence means that intimacy becomes altogether too dangerous, and as with so many other aspects of life, it slowly becomes the business of professionals to manufacture a marketable substitute for it. More and more the hazardous birth of undefended intimacy between people is seen as needing to be attended by professional midwives of some description, and people are taught the ritual 'skills' which are supposed to ensure safe and 'meaningful' relationship. In an increasingly wide range of settings – from evening classes to church congregations – lonely people are propelled into a mutually self-deceiving 'togetherness' by means of superficial 'techniques' and games (e.g. 'ice-breakers') which are claimed by their professional inventors to be the answer to our 'alienation'. Instant intimacy becomes something you can buy from your local encounter group centre.

When people have nothing other than themselves to talk about,

conversations become parallel monologues in which the participants take turns to recite their likes and dislikes, complain or
make confessions which (because of the 'no criticism' pact) are
guaranteed a blandly tolerant hearing. Groups or congregations of
people who are aware of their own or others' isolation become for
want of any real activity artificially (semi-professionally)
constructed round a collaborative contemplation of self, with the
result that the group soon finds itself enmired in utterly futile
discussions of how its members 'relate to' each other – as though
'relating' were a special and specific kind of activity which people
can do.

There is something very sad and touching about our frustrated
need for companionship. Though it is not a fashionable view, and
is one rejected by most of those whose opinions I respect (as well
as espoused by some whose opinions I do not), I do have a sneaking
feeling that, given half a chance, most people would treat their
fellows reasonably decently. The almost desperate love which
people lavish on their dogs, for example, leads one to wonder how
basic to human *nature* human cruelty is. Might it not rather be
that the kinds of threat to which we respond so violently and
brutally are built into our society more than into our selves? If the
sheer scale of our inhumanity towards each other to which both
our history and our current conduct and experience testify is to be
taken as an indication of the depth of some kind of original sin or
ineradicable natural trait, we might as well consign our species to
an atomic oblivion forthwith. It does appear to me, though, that
many of those who have been lovingly cared for care lovingly for
others, and that many of those who cause pain and injury to others
do so out of a kind of anguished blindness born of circumstances
which they could not escape rather than of any kind of ill-will
or avoidable impulse. Unquestionably there is the most appalling
violence built into the structure of our society (its hierarchical
inequality could be maintained no other way), but the more intimately I get to know those (i.e. all of us) who are the agents of
that violence, the less easy I find it to identify things *within them*
to blame.

Without doubt, many of the people I have worked with who
have been badly damaged through their relations with others have
been or are being equally damaging *to* others, but from the un-
threatened – and hence I think more clear-sighted – position of
psychotherapist, that has not made them any harder to understand
or like. For example, one watches people struggle in vain not to
make their children insecure, or listens to a young couple recount
with uncomprehending hopelessness how their baby died through
their neglect, and all one can feel is a kind of helpless sympathy.

The reasons for the violence we do each other are all too clear, but do not reside in the individual agent. This insight – common, I think, to many of those who work in the 'helping professions' even if they do not always make it explicit – is one which renders particularly repugnant the righteous indignation of those who pontificate about the state of public morality, and utterly disgusting the 'media's' baying for the punishment of people whose wretchedness leads to tragedy.

Given a safe enough environment, then, it seems to me that most people are glad of an opportunity to love their fellows. The travesty of friendship which one sees in our rituals of fake intimacy, the timid confidences which are barely heard by partners absorbed in the formulation of what they intend to confide in their turn, indicate an altruism stunted and frustrated by a society which dislocates people from a world of constructive action and turns them against each other in bitter competition. If we do not truly 'open up' to each other, 'be sensitive', 'show our feelings' in the way that the therapy industry encourages us to do, it is because we have good reasons not to – we live in a social world which really is dangerous. To try to solve the 'problem' by, again, manipulating the surface phenomena of individual behaviour (i.e. simulating behavioural effects rather than tackling socio-economic causes), is to foster just the kind of faking and artificiality with which we are so familiar from the world of 'marketing' and to ignore the abuses of power which underlie our rational fear and suspicion of each other.

On the evidence to date, it would stretch credulity beyond all reasonable limits to suggest that human beings, or human society, were truly perfectible in any absolute sense, and I do not want to lay claim to a vision of a utopian world in which sweetness and light will reign supreme and undisturbed. One need not lapse into 'biologisms' concerning human 'nature' or 'instincts' to observe the hair-trigger nervousness and violence with which people and societies react to threat,* and the quite appalling terror and oppression which they will resort to in establishing and protecting their interests. But however inevitable much of this may be there is still enormous room for improvement, and such improvement can only sensibly be looked for in the social, moral and political

---

*Interesting treatments of the question of violence and destructiveness are to be found in, for example, E. Fromm, *The Anatomy of Human Destructiveness*, Penguin Books, 1977, and F. Wertham, *A Sign for Cain. An Exploration of Human Violence*, Hale, 1966. It is inevitable that such books raise questions rather than provide answers, but these at least raise interesting questions.

spheres. Individual consciousness and relations between individuals reflect rather than cause the power structure within society. In situations where threat is absent or minimized (there can be very few of these – the nearest I can think of are some of the artificially constructed 'therapeutic communities' which were created in the sixties for the treatment of 'mental illness'*) or where people are united in opposition to a *common* threat (as in war), people do seem to be able to conduct themselves towards each other with concern, interest and affection.

Concern, interest and affection are becoming precisely those characteristics of relationship which have to be either faked or bartered. We have an awareness of each other's neediness, but the latter is so great that we have to make special arrangements for its (very partial) fulfilment, which is either bought from professionals, carefully shared out in parallel conversations in which turns are taken at self-revelation, or merely simulated in ritual but empty gestures of intimacy (e.g. the technology of the 'encounter' group).

Sex

It has become almost impossible to think clearly or constructively about sex, since sexual satisfaction is the pivot around which our commercial culture turns, the sacred central axiom of a dogma of gratification which will not allow itself to be questioned or criticized. To suggest, for instance, that sex should be *for* anything other than itself, or to speculate that there could be *any* grounds for control of or abstinence from sexual indulgence (even, for example, in order to avoid a risk of fatal disease) is to invite immediate dismissal from the community of rational beings, even to occasion worried concern for the state of one's mental health. The isolation of sex from procreation and the refinement and promulgation of sexual pleasures of every form and variety, the 'liberation' of women by the pill and the widespread acceptance and endorsement of forms of sexuality once considered 'perverse', all these are seen as the triumphs of an age which has freed us from sexual prudery, repression and hypocrisy, and given us permission to pursue our pleasures, to explore and exploit each other's orifices without a shred of shame.

Let me hasten to reassure the reader at this point that I am not about to advocate a 'return' to no-doubt mythical standards of a past sexual propriety, to suggest that we abandon contraception, impose unnecessary abstinence upon ourselves or make homosexu-

*See D. Kennard, *An Introduction to Therapeutic Communities*, Routledge and Kegan Paul, 1983.

ality illegal. What we do need to do, however, is to restore to sexuality a meaning, to re-embed it in our personal lives and relations such that it regains significances beyond itself.

In his book *The History of Sexuality*,* Michel Foucault suggests that the nineteenth century, far from being an era of sexual repression, was one when sex in fact became the focus of attention, discussion and scientific investigation as never before. And indeed it does seem to be the case that in the course of the past hundred years or so, and with a rapid acceleration in very recent decades, sexuality has been torn out of any kind of context to be presented before us as the absolute raw material of gratification; sex becomes as inherently meaningless but as essentially important to personal survival and satisfaction as money, and, like money, it is attached to both people and things – commodities – to lend them a certain kind of value.

Dislodged from the spatial context of the embodied relations of men and women, as well as from the temporal context of our personal histories, sex is installed as the irreducible absolute at the centre of a commercialized religion of satisfaction, and to ask questions about its meaning and its value is to commit a kind of blasphemy. Where once sex may have been surrounded by a moralism of prudish disapproval, it is now hedged about with, if anything, an even more thornily impenetrable if quite different moralism, i.e. one which permits no challenge to the creed that everyone shall be permitted to enjoy themselves in any way they choose – 'whatever turns you on'.

The main reason for sexual pleasure's having come to occupy this central and unassailable position as a kind of cultural imperative is, I suspect, because of its extraordinary efficacy in selling things. Whether or not Freud was right to make 'libido' the foundation of human psychology, there seems little doubt that sexual energy has become the basic fuel of the commercial interests which structure our society. We are sold 'happiness' and 'satisfaction' by an appeal to their crudest and most basic 'fulfilment', and it seems as though organizations and institutions at virtually every level of society conspire progressively to loosen us from any restraint we may feel in giving the fullest rein to sexual indulgence. Industry, advertising, education, health, therapy and counselling combine to give us the green light to pursue gratification to the utmost, to douse in any way we dream up the nervous itch of our desires.

Sex is a marvellous medium for commodity sales in a market which demands infinite expansion and the endless obsolescence of

*Published by Penguin Books in 1981. The title is somewhat misleading in the light of the original French, *La Volonté de Savoir*.

fashion, for no sooner has the nervous system achieved a blissful sexual peace than the engine starts once more to hum, and before you know where you are the cycle starts all over again. There is, it is true, an overall element of satiation in this process which necessitates a continuous escalation in the stimulation of desire, so that appeals to the 'joy of sex' need, step by step, to be made ever coarser and more direct. (Where once the camera dwelt shyly on knees, it now stares straight into the crutch.) But presumably there is still considerable mileage left in sex.

I do not wish to say that we have become a society of sex maniacs, or to expostulate indignantly about our 'shame', but only to suggest that what we take to be liberation may be in fact enslavement. For the pursuit of sexual gratification seems to be doing very little for 'relationships', and couples seem to become increasingly split and isolated from one another as each partner concentrates anxiously on his technique, worries obsessively about her attractiveness, and assesses self-consciously the scale of his or her satisfaction. Indeed, it seems to have become for many people a source of irritation that they have to depend on someone else to meet their sexual needs, and when not actually in bed, men and women tend to eye each other with hostility and contempt, secretly promising themselves an exchange of partner as soon as a more satisfactory 'relationship' appears, reluctantly and frustratedly settling for what they have got when it no longer seems that it is going to. As with 'relationship' itself, sex has become the commodity of which people are the interchangeable vehicles, anonymous purveyors of reassurance or an ego-boost, a momentary respite from sexual restlessness. We use each other to satisfy needs so personal as to be almost autistic, and sex becomes a kind of suspicious bartering of incompatible self-indulgences rather than the unifying joy which sexual rhetoric proclaims. This situation is epitomized in the 'sex therapy' industry, which advocates a technicized exchange of gratifications whose 'demandingness' may be carefully graded and controlled.

Although I have no doubt that it would be going much too far to suggest that sexual love has become entirely an outdated romantic notion, it does seem to me that, though people may expect and long for 'deeply fulfilling' sexual relationships, what for the most part they actually find are uncomfortably combative liaisons of the kind I have outlined above. The reason for this, once again, is to be sought not inside individuals, but may be traced to the nature of our society. As well as being split off by commercial interests from any relational meaning (sex no longer arises from a relation to a *particular person*, but, like 'consumer durables', is a product to which the agents of production are irrelevant), sexuality is located in a social context in which men and women confront each other in a spirit of competition. In a brave and brilliant book* which I imagine must, despite its artistry, have lost him a good deal of support among 'conventional' feminists and other critics of contemporary society, Ivan Illich has suggested that an economy which engineers competition for goods and resources perceived as scarce, encourages men and women to conduct themselves as beings of essentially the *same kind*, apart from an accidental difference in sex, who must compete uniformly for the goods and services on offer. In this way we become what Illich calls 'sexed neuters', stripped of any kind of complementary gender, and distinguishable from each other only by the 'bulge in the blue jeans'. As more and more of the traditional fields of 'gendered' work and activity are thrown into the modern unisex economy – for example as men begin to concern themselves with the arts of baby care – so the battle-ground of hostile competition between men and women is widened. 'Invidious comparison now replaces awe as the reaction to otherness.'

In almost everything one hears or reads, those 'sexual partners' who are not simply burying their emotions in some kind of wishful mythology seem to be asking themselves where they went wrong, or hurrying from the bloody wreckage of the last 'relationship' to peer hopefully round the corner to see if the next one looks more promising. But we are caught up in processes beyond our selves and our individual strengths and weaknesses. Once again, it has to be pointed out that we cannot escape (unless completely artificially) the ground we stand on and the air we breathe: relations between men and women have been cast into confusion by forces beyond their control, and consequently the experience and meaning of sex – apart from its commodity value – has also been thrown into question.

It seems unlikely that the solution to this predicament can lie in some artificial form of retrogression to a time when men and women accepted (however unjustly) roles in society which were gendered and complementary. Rather, we are confronted with a situation in which the nineteenth-century psychological myth of the primacy of sex is peeling away to reveal a 'more primary' issue of power, and how that issue will be resolved only time will tell.

Sex, if ever it was, is no longer a matter for repression, but questions concerning power and interest are, and our, as it were, cultural assertion of the absolute value of sexual pleasure makes it surprisingly difficult to inquire into the history and phenomenology of power which seem to lurk behind and within the difficulties

* I. Illich, *Gender*, Marion Boyars, 1983.

people experience and the injuries they inflict on each other in their sexual encounters. There is an enormous contrast between the images of sexual satisfaction in which our culture trades and the actual experience of the people who are subjected to them, but attempts to *explicate* sexual experience (rather than to tend it or stoke it 'therapeutically') are quite often met with refusal or even anger. But, I suspect, if one is to gain any understanding of the painful strife which so often these days infuses both hetero- and homosexual relations, one will have to be prepared to trace them back into the power relations which society imposes on its members. In this way, the sexual experience and proclivities of individuals cannot be fully understood without investigating their personal history, particularly in terms of the permutations of relations between mothers and fathers and sons and daughters, since it is through these relations that the wider social influences make themselves felt. Inevitably, *we* are the agents of our society's exploitation, and the most potent source of learning in the ways of relationship (for good or for ill) is the family. The purpose of trying to trace, for example, the significance of (among other things) individuals' sexual conduct back into their personal histories is not, as will be evident from the previous chapter, to seek to change it, but rather to develop the beginnings of an understanding of how we come to shape our children in ways of relationship which they cannot escape.

Marriage

For the psychologist (or anyone else) interested in the kinds of 'relationship' which seem so to preoccupy us, marriage provides the magnifying glass through which they may be most closely studied, for it is in the (relatively) long-term contract of marriage that our mythical expectations as well as our actual experience of 'relationship' are most clearly exposed.

More than any other form of relationship, marriage carries our hopes for a warm, fulfilling, safe, confiding, mentally and physically satisfying bond with another person. Yet in practice marriage causes more bitterness, resentment, disappointment and inarticulate pain than all our other 'relationships' put together. For countless people, what is confidently embarked upon as an exclusive mutual alliance against an indifferent or hostile world, a search for a haven of warmth in a cold and competitive society, turns out to be a journey into a totally unexpected, private and unanalysable hell – one seeming, furthermore, to constitute an entirely personal and exceptional misery which, if it is not ended in a burst of hatred and recrimination, can only be endured with dumb incomprehension.

I do not wish either to decry or to discredit the institution of marriage, and I have no doubt that for many people (though, if they are honest, I suspect not unequivocally) it does provide a refuge of warmth and support without which they would find emotional survival extremely difficult. However, I do not believe that this can be the best or most creative function of marriage: if our world is so beastly that we need to escape from it into the comparative safety of an isolated pact with one other person, we need to indict the world rather than extol marriage. It is in any case almost impossible to gain a clear view of marriage through the haze of wishful fantasy which surrounds it and which, as ever, is endlessly and relentlessly fuelled by commercial interests. In modern marriage, we have been overtaken by a phenomenon of relationship of which we have no sober or reflective understanding, but only the wildest and most unrealistic expectations. To be able to spend forty or more years living happily, or merely reasonably comfortably, with a single partner – even, or perhaps especially, if bonded initially by intense sexual desire – is one of the most testing demands people can place upon themselves, and it is thus small wonder that attitudes generated by the experience of marriage tend to split between cynical dismissal and self-deluding sentimentality. Neither of these extremes seems appropriate to me: precisely because marriage is so central to our social structure, and yet so demanding and so much a source of pain and bewilderment, it seems to me that our stance towards it should be one of honesty and respect. We need to gain an accurate and honest appreciation of the emotional demands of marriage and to develop a sober assessment of what marriage may be *for* if it is not to be simply *for itself* in the sense of constituting the ultimate in gratifying and fulfilling 'relationships'. Above all, I think, we need to illuminate the men and women who stand at either term of the marriage 'relationship', i.e. to 'de-commodify' the relationship and to discover the people who are so easily sacrificed in its pursuit and who suffer so bitterly as the result. Respect for the extraordinary difficulty entailed by marriage may lead to respect for the partners who enter into it. If it is not to disintegrate in reciprocal hatred or become submerged in a deadening sentimental banality, marriage cannot be expected to be an end in itself, a pact of mutual self-indulgence, but must be recognized as a kind of commitment partners make to each other *for* something beyond the commitment itself and the 'happiness' it is (falsely) expected to generate. It may of course turn out to be the case that in the modern world there is nothing much other than itself which marriage can be for. In which case, we may safely expect its gradual demise as an institution.

Up until comparatively very recent times marriage was linked much more clearly to economic necessity and the social power structure than to the search for blissful 'relationship'. As Lawrence Stone points out,* the 'companionate marriage' was largely a creation of the eighteenth century, by which time many of the socio-economic, contractual reasons for marriage had diminished, leaving an increasingly individualistic and pleasure-seeking middle and upper class in pursuit of forms of happiness for which the still officially indissoluble bond of marriage offered to provide a ready receptacle. Furthermore, it is only even more recently that marriage can be almost relied upon to last a lifetime (hence, Stone argues, our need for divorce to perform the task more frequently performed before by death). From serving hard-headed and practical interests, then, marriage came to serve as a kind of private personal indulgence, the satisfaction of needs for emotional comfort and companionship.

The romanticizing of love and marriage in this way had dangers which were not lost on observers of the time. Stone quotes Oliver Goldsmith's warning concerning the 'mystification' of marriage:

> How delusive, how destructive, are those pictures of consummate bliss. They teach the youthful mind to sigh after beauty and happiness which never existed, to despise that little good which fortune has mixed up in our cup, by expecting more than she ever gave.

However, Stone's work also suggests that changes in the social structure in which marriage is embedded, giving rise as they did to the 'companionate marriage', led concomitantly to generally more gentle and affectionate relations within families and to a greater interest than hitherto in questions of education and child welfare, so perhaps it would be ungracious to dismiss too quickly as mere self-indulgence any indication of social movement towards a climate of opinion which begins to take seriously the well-being of others. Perhaps, again, this was one of those points in history where, in another context, enlightened and altruistic thought (for example like that of Rousseau) might have led to a sustained improvement in social conditions generally. However, nothing demonstrates more clearly than the career of our attitude to marriage the pervasiveness of the corruption of interest. For, as with sex, the comforts and consolations of 'companionate'

*L. Stone, *The Family, Sex and Marriage in England 1500–1800*, Penguin Books, 1979.

marriage have been commercially isolated and magnified, infused with our greedy fantasies and served up to us as a 'package' at once so attractive and so illusory that we can scarcely any longer bring to bear upon it any form of coherent criticism.* Whatever else may be the case, it certainly seems that the 'affective individualism' of which Stone writes has arrived in our own time at a point where any possibility of our being meaningfully related to a social world outside ourselves has become, as it were, imploded into an intensely focused 'relationship' which is expected to be not only 'companionate', but even therapeutic, not only sexually fulfilling, but self-sufficiently and completely emotionally gratifying. If we continue on this course, there is, saving death itself, only one more stop on the way to our destination, and that is complete individual self-sufficiency; the ultimate in security is being able to do without *anyone*.

There is virtually nothing in, on the one hand, the welter of sentimentality, mythology and wishful thinking, and on the other the angry disillusion surrounding marriage, by which we may begin to make sense of our experience of married life. Over and over again people run up against completely unexpected obstacles to their continued marital happiness from which they recoil hurt and bewildered, believing themselves in an entirely individual predicament which must be put down to someone's 'fault' – either their partner's or their own. The irony is that this is in fact the almost inevitable fate of all those 'embodied subjects' who find themselves located in this particular world.

There are three particularly frequent constellations of marital difficulty which may be taken as examples of what I mean. They correspond roughly to what may be expected (when troubles do arise) in the early, middle and later stages of marriage, and might be termed accordingly the phases of disillusion, re-illusion and resignation.

The disillusion of early marriage is, despite its near-universality, experienced by those it affects usually silently and very privately, as a particularly unfortunate and personal failing. As the absorp-

---

*A characteristically honest (if almost brutally sour!) antidote to the kind of false sentimentality concerning marriage which is so evident in popular literature is provided by Leo Tolstoy in an observation in his diary for 30 August 1894: 'Novels end with the hero and heroine getting married. They should begin with that and end with them getting unmarried, i.e. becoming free. Otherwise to describe people's lives in such a way as to break off the description with marriage is just the same as describing a person's journey and breaking off the description at the point where the traveller falls into the hands of robbers.' (*Tolstoy's Diaries*, Vol. I, edited by R. F. Christian, Athlone Press, 1985.)

tion in each other wears away and the exigencies of the world outside 'the relationship' begin to reassert themselves, each partner reads in the conduct of the other a personal betrayal, or in their own disappointment a shameful failure of commitment. The husband (to take the still typical case) finds his wife's lack of understanding for the call on his attention of his work commitments, and her demand for continual demonstration of his interest in and affection towards her, irksome and unfair – can't she *see* how much he thinks of her? Can't she tell that the work he does is for her (and perhaps for their young children)? Can't she see that he needs to relax when he gets home, not to talk about a day he wants to forget, nor to hear the trivial details of hers? These feelings his wife interprets as a treacherous decrease of the loving involvement he had shown. He no longer seems to care, and all she experiences is the enervating isolation of a life incarcerated with small children, few friends and a family she rarely sees. Her husband is uncommunicative, elsewhere, absorbed in a world of power and money (even if only at the very bottom of its hierarchy) which seems to mean more to him than she. They no longer talk to each other as they did. He gets more out of talking to the people who share his working world, she makes a confidante of one or two young mothers she knows. She feels his sexual interest in her as invasive and insincere, mere lust. He is hurt and bewildered by her lessened sexual interest in him. Each feels that 'the marriage' threatens to be a failure; it is not what it was, and has not turned out either as they expected or as it should. Perhaps they were, after all, not right for each other.

And so to the phase of re-illusion, in which the partners cast around to rediscover what they feel they have lost. For the wife, busy with tending to the needs of children, this may mean little more than daydreaming, fantasizing the appearance of a kind and attentive, gentle man who will love her for herself alone. As long as she is dependent on her husband for her keep, she can afford to show him little of these feelings, but if she becomes more financially independent as the children get older, she may begin to allow her contempt and resentment to show rather more boldly; perhaps also she will turn the children into partners in an alliance against the unfeeling and insensitive male, the father/husband whose still too-powerful figure begins to throw a shadow almost of dread over the household. Re-illusion is perhaps particularly the province of the male. The husband, sexually rejected, hurt and perhaps excluded (though perhaps none of these, but rather just pining for the lost adulation of a woman) finds himself embroiled in a 'relationship' with another woman – the disillusioned wife of a friend, possibly, or a younger unattached woman at work. The springtime of his life miraculously reappears – it *is* possible to be loved! And so, confident in the belief perhaps that he now knows enough from his experience of life *really* to make 'the relationship' work, off he goes with his new-found love to start the cycle all over again, leaving at home a woman too old, too tired, too encumbered with children and far too angry to be very likely to take a similar course.

Resignation comes when you look up after fifteen or so years of child-rearing to find yourself sharing a lonely life with a hostile stranger. Darby and Joan bickering and sniping at each other with practised weariness. Far from finding their lives a cosy therapeutic oneness, they tolerate each other's presence filled with a kind of seething irritation in which their all-too-familiar mannerisms, even the rustle of their clothes or the sound of their breathing, are enough to trigger in the other a barely suppressed wave of frustrated rage. For simply sharing a home and a family does not automatically lead to unity of soul and body – indeed many people could probably more easily share their declining years with a workmate of long standing than with a spouse. Partners' concerns and interests diverge over time more often than they converge, and the second half of life – particularly perhaps for women who have invested a great deal in now fully fledged children – can plunge people into a sense of isolation and despairing futility at once inescapable and totally unexpected. Professional guidance and 'the media' as well as popular literature and entertainment all emphasize the positive value of 'relationships' and proffer a technology for making them 'work'. For this reason it is often with stunned bewilderment that people come face to face with their predicament. *Nothing* prepares us for the difficulties of marriage in a world which imposes on people the way, in what roles and arenas, they shall live their lives. The end is resignation, the discovery that, after all, you have been cheated of happiness, and can only wait for death in a state of armed truce with your 'one and only'. But your disappointment will be of no concern to society as a whole, as by now you have lost your economic significance. The advertisement, like all advertisements, turns out in the end to be a lie, but no one will mind, since you will have spent as much on the product as you can be expected to.

To look at the way we treat the elderly with a gaze as far as possible unclouded by custom and practice – as if newly arrived from some other planet where they order things better – is to be overcome with horror. These are not people sustained by years of therapeutic relationship, but rather people no longer serving the purposes that never were their own – no longer serving any purpose at all.

I should probably emphasize once more at this point that what I want to draw attention to are the constraints placed upon our lives by the structure of the society in which we live and the mythology which has become established in its service. I have known enough people who, sometimes in the face of almost unimaginable adversity, live their lives with the greatest concern for and commitment to those they share it with, not lightly to devalue their undertaking. My intention is not cynically to disparage the loving concern many people still, against all the odds, manage to show to others, including their spouses, but rather to attack the values of a society which makes preparation for and understanding of 'relationship' so difficult and successful 'relatedness' so rare.

We need in fact to dismantle the mystifying rhetoric of 'relationship' which, in order to sell us a whole range of illusory satisfactions and to maintain us in isolated, inactive and uncomplaining battery units, promises us total gratification in blissful union with our loved one, and to construct instead a realistic appreciation of what a commitment to other people must entail. It seems obvious, for example, that to found the happiness of one's life on another *person* is to lay upon him or her a strain which the human spirit is just too weak to bear, and for two people who are historically and organically different from each other to be expected to provide a *mutually* supportive programme of more or less therapeutic 'understanding' and emotional tolerance, not to mention sexual indulgence, is stretching the bounds of possibility beyond all reasonable limit. As far as this is our expectation of marriage it is bound to be disappointed. The task of couples who wish both to stay married and to maintain some kind of contact with reality must be to learn to accept in the self and permit (and tolerate) in the other an inevitable degree of isolation and 'difference'. There must be, as it were, permissible areas of non-understanding, recognition of untouchable and impenetrable uniqueness, preparedness to enter some experiences entirely alone and unaided by emotional support, not because such support is being wilfully withheld (and might be available in a 'better' relationship) but because its supply is illusory. This calls for a tolerance of pain, and an understanding of its nature, which few of us these days are able to command. Each partner needs to see in the other a man or woman with needs, weaknesses, fears and idiosyncrasies parallel to (though far from identical with) his or her own, not the more or less adequate purveyor, or indeed recipient, of satisfactions – 'love' and 'understanding' – which are the stuff of commodified relationship.

If, of course, marriage is an end in itself, a bid for emotional security in an otherwise hostile world, the kind of tolerance of difference I am advocating would amount to an entirely unacceptable renunciation of bliss. But precisely because of the impossible demands marriage-for-itself places on its partners, I do not believe that it can survive as such. It is easy enough to see what marriage has been *for* in the past (economic advantage or security, the forging of familial alliances, etc.), but less easy to see what form it may take in the future. If, however, we come to acknowledge that 'relationships' of all kinds can arise meaningfully only from being for something other than themselves, there is no reason why marriage should not continue as an institution 'for' something. Even now, it may legitimately enough be seen as for the rearing of children.

Parents and Children

The way in which the human body is constructed makes it certain that power will arise as a central issue in human life, and the way in which human society is organized will determine how power is to be distributed, used or abused. Inevitably, some people are stronger than others – men (on the whole) than women, adults (always) than infants. It is for this basic and obvious reason that at the very root of the inequality of our power-infused social hierarchy are to be found violence and the threat of violence (terror). Nowhere is the issue of power more salient than in the relations between parents and children, and nowhere are its roots in violence and terror more frequently, and sadly, exposed.

I find it a matter of some considerable surprise that psychologists, and especially those clinically involved in the study and 'treatment' of families, have not thought about and addressed more centrally the issue of power. It has not, certainly, been totally absent from the thinking of some psychologists, especially those interested in people's social relations more than merely in their internal psychic workings – one thinks, for example, of Alfred Adler and those influenced by him – but on the whole the issue of power has been overshadowed by, one might say hidden behind, that of sex, and there seems little doubt that Freud's influence in this has been enormous. It is tempting to think that concern with the 'repression' of sexuality which Freud and his colleagues worked so assiduously to lift served, however unintendedly, as a screen for a much deeper and more pervasive repression – that of power, its inequalities and injustices. For if, as Foucault argues, sexuality was far from being the taboo subject (and practice) of Victorian society which we have been led to believe, it was precisely in this period of European history and colonial domination (not to mention familial relations) that the oppressive use of power reached unprecedented heights of organization and sophistication. It is, again, surprising

113

that, despite the resistance Freud felt he encountered (and resented so bitterly) towards his theories, his ideas on sexuality were in fact accepted almost eagerly and adopted into twentieth-century culture with great rapidity, when even now one might expect them to stretch the credulity of an averagely critical mind beyond the normal bounds of reason. And yet at the same time, the quite obvious importance of disparities in power between adults and children was largely ignored, and indeed it still is ignored by most of us today. The basest of human motives lie not in our sexual affiliations, but in our violence towards one another, and it is above all these motives which we repress most effectively.

In the orthodox view of the 'Oedipus complex', for example, the power struggle between son and father is treated in psychoanalytic thinking as secondary to a sexual struggle for the mother/wife. I must confess that I have always had difficulty in being able to take seriously the psychoanalytic view of sexuality in infancy and childhood, not least because I have never been struck, as psychoanalysts clearly seem to be, by a particularly significant sexual component even to the most honest and undefended accounts people give of their childhood experience, nor have I observed any particularly potent or impressive sexual activities or impulses in pre-pubertal children (which is not to say that such children are innocent of all sexual feeling or conduct, nor that they may not imitate sexually mature activity). I have, of course, come across very powerful and often very destructive sexual components in the relations of adults *towards* children, not infrequently their own, but this is of course quite another matter. Competition between parents for the alliance of their children is very often observable and frequently not without elements of sexual seductiveness. In this way a renaming of the 'Oedipus complex' as the 'Jocasta complex' (after Oedipus's mother) would make a kind of psychological sense more often supported by actual clinical experience: mothers who seduce their sons (and none the less powerfully for being only metaphorically) in order to isolate and in a sense castrate their husbands are a far from rare phenomenon (and certainly have a part to play in the genesis of male homosexuality) – but here again the essential theme, the key to the understanding of the 'dynamics', is one of *power*. Though, of course, a small child can play on the weaknesses of its parents and so exploit their differences, its power in such situations is merely passive or negative; its resources of positive power are, in relation to those of its parents, negligible.

Sons struggle against paternal domination; fathers crush, tyrannize or patronize daughters; mothers manoeuvre fairly or foully against male oppression, monopolize their sons' affection or competitively drain their daughters of female competence in exactly the way that a father can use his power never to allow his son to surpass him in anything. The 'pathology' of family relations knows many permutations and variations, but most centre on the misuse, abuse and fear of power. One can very often detect, even on quite casual acquaintance, how people have learned to deal with their earliest experiences of the power of others. In the way, for example, that they characteristically try to assert their own interests – charmingly, perhaps, or cajolingly, defiantly, fearfully, obliquely, seductively, angrily, sullenly, insistently, etc., etc. – one can almost see the shadow of a parent falling over them.

We have not developed very much in the way of an ethics of child-rearing in our culture, and the very idea that we should give much thought to what might be good for our children seems, in modern times at least, to have struck us as at all significant only since the eighteenth century.* We have yet to meditate seriously on the *overwhelming* disparity of power between adults and children (though, of course, we do not hesitate to make remorseless use of it) and where we do get a glimpse of the ravages the powerful (adults) wreak on the powerless (children) our first – and so far only – thought seems to be to 'disband' the family and seek other ways of organizing the basic units of society. However, nothing will eradicate the disparity of power between adults and children, and we might, rather than trying to get rid of it, attempt to find ways of using it for good rather than ill.

Once again we have at present no concepts even to begin to think about this undertaking other than those of a semi-articulated authoritarian moralism or various forms of laissez-faire. This, I think, is because of the extent of the repression of power in the wider society. Because we do not comment about or reflect upon injustice and inequality to any really serious degree, because we are all to some extent involved in turning blind eyes to the free play of violence and exploitation in the pursuit of interest, we can only watch helplessly as these forms of relation reproduce themselves within our families.

It is not that parents harbour any evil intent towards their children, and it is the cruellest of errors to suppose that they do by, for example, dragging the concept of blame into a consideration of who causes whom psychological injury or distress. It is rather that, in a culture in which we have no articulate conception of the loving use of power (and if we ever had one in the past we have lost it), we are thrown together in contexts – as for example

*L. Stone, op. cit. See also Phillipe Ariès, *Centuries of Childhood*, Jonathan Cape, 1962.

families – in which our relations are going inevitably to be shaped by the social forms of the wider environment.

I do not think it any exaggeration to say that we are approaching a state of affairs in which we simply do not know how to relate to one another except coercively and exploitingly, and the effects of this are going to be particularly severe in cases where – as between children and adults – there are gross disparities in power. My reasons for feeling this are based on no mere abstract consideration of social speculation or political theory, but on the endlessly and dishearteningly repeated experience of witnessing the deformation and ineradicable emotional scarring of people who were once children by parents whose only conscious wish was to love them.

At a relatively coarse level of analysis, there are several almost standard ways – familiar, I would suggest, in most people's experience – in which the fundamentally baleful nature of our society is reflected in the manner in which parental power comes to be exerted over children. Without running into further volumes, I can do no more here than sketch some of them rather as caricatures.

At the bottom of the pyramid, the very base of the social hierarchy, many people are just too drained and oppressed, too robbed of ability or initiative to feel that they can or want to do anything for their children but simply to keep them quiet. In this kind of situation children are likely to be indulged, neglected, bullied or mistreated, handed over to 'experts' in the welfare services, and generally left to find their way through the system as best they can. Nobody will have the resources of time, money or personal concern to observe their talents or nurture their interests and abilities, though they may encounter a degree of formal (but, because overstretched, highly undependable) support from official agencies. To avoid becoming nothing more than fodder for a depressed labour market or marginally useful for the consumption of mass-produced junk, the child in this position needs an almost miraculously lucky encounter with someone (most often an unusually strong and capable grandparent or aunt or uncle) who will through his or her affection, wisdom and energy, open up for it a world of possibility and a realization of its own potentialities which would otherwise be missed. The only consolation to occupancy of this level of society, and it is indeed the smallest of mercies, is that tired neglect, though it generates the most dreadful waste, often avoids the malign distortion of growth which leads to such emotional pain in people who have been subjected to more positive abuses of power.

It is virtually impossible to occupy a precariously insecure position in the power hierarchy without the anxiety and hostility such a position occasions being reflected in family relations. People who, as it were, find themselves perched on a ledge a little way up the social pyramid – far enough to want desperately to hang on to the small advantage gained but not far enough to be unaware of the unattractiveness of rock bottom – live particularly threatened lives, and it can be little surprise if they hedge their children round with all kinds of exhortations and prohibitions, keen for them to climb higher and anxious lest they drag the family back down to what they see as social ignominy. Here is to be found the much maligned 'petty bourgeoisie', renowned for its mean-spirited narrow-mindedness, envy and authoritarian moralism. But the values of generosity and liberalism make little sense to anyone having to cling to this perch, where the threat of economic power is probably felt at its most acute and life becomes an unrelenting pursuit of an always just-unattainable security, a panicky clinging to advantages gained and an angry contempt both for people who have silver spoons in their mouths and for those who have fallen back into torpid resignation. The reality here is of economic survival and obedient subservience to power, and other values, other ways of perceiving the world, become mere self-indulgence. Rigid conformity to narrowly ideal standards and denial and repression of emotions, perceptions and values which do not meet them, resentful respect for authority and uncritical acceptance of established social institutions breed an atmosphere in which children are likely to find it hard to develop a firm sense of subjectivity, but will be moulded to occupancy of stereotyped social and sexual roles and will experience considerable anxiety and guilt when they find themselves departing from them. Self-deception and hypocrisy, emotional deprivation and defensiveness follow naturally from this kind of situation, which, not surprisingly, is one of the most psychologically mutilating in which one can find oneself.

It is in this stratum, and those close to it, that the course of development most typical of our society is perhaps most obviously to be found – the transformation of a lively and promising human infant, through a period of indoctrination, disillusion and rebellion, into an emotionally constricted, competitively hostile adult saturated in the values of commodity consumption, desperately conforming, anxiously pursuing an ever-receding 'happiness', bereft of any ability to criticize the society in which he or she is located, pathetically eager to enjoy those of its 'fruits' (consumer durables) which are within reach. This is the great, inertially stable backbone of our society, the guardian of its values and the target of its mass media, working tirelessly in the interests of others and blindly against its own, forced by the crushing vice of economic power into reproducing itself reliably and endlessly in its children.

At the upper level of this stratum, and extending into the managerial and professional strata, one finds family relations set in a rather less rigid context in which a degree of economic security allows room for, on the one hand, genuinely realizable ambition, and on the other economically riskable (though strictly one-dimensional*) criticism of the *status quo*. Here, for example, managers may manage their children, organizing their experience (e.g. controlling what television programmes may be watched) and to a lesser extent their social and educational environment in accordance with aims seen as desirable and attainable. The relatively greater degree of power available at this level makes in general for a rather more relaxed and less moralistic hedonism, but the culture is still likely to be highly materialistic in one form or another and the emphasis in child-rearing will probably be on the gaining of increased status, so that children will often experience strong pressure to achieve and 'succeed'. In the absence of crude economic threat (e.g. relative security of parental job tenure and provision of pensions, etc.), the atmosphere is more often likely to be one of alienation rather than anxiety: the pursuit of comfort and satisfaction, the possibility of actually obtaining recurrent quiescence of the nervous system, may lead to a kind of flaccidity in values, an incipient sense of purposelessness and a desperation to realize purpose in 'relationships', which result in fact in chaotic, manipulative and dishonest relations between parents. Children in this type of situation may be or feel emotionally distanced from their families, and their parents, intent on pursuing their own gratification, may simply buy their offspring's upbringing from educationalists and 'experts' of one sort or another. Particularly in the families of middle-class intellectuals and academics children may be permitted or actually encouraged a kind of rebellion against conventional norms as long as they 'achieve' intellectually. In adolescents from this kind of background one can often encounter an intelligent criticism of their parents' apparently dishonest involvement in materialist values and lack of emotional commitment to anything very much, but idealism seems to give way all too soon to a learned indifference to people, a sort of profound disaffection which in the end simply reproduces a drifting indulgence in commodified relationships and embarkation on one of society's more comfortable vocational bandwagons, propelled more by fashion than commitment.

*I mean this in the sense developed by Herbert Marcuse in *One-Dimensional Man*, Beacon Press, 1964, i.e. that criticism of the social and conceptual *status quo* is possible only in the forms and language prescribed by the self-same *status quo*, and hence never challenges its fundamental values.

It is only perhaps towards the apex of the social hierarchy that one any longer comes across the most direct application of economic power within the family itself, i.e. the parental control of children through the straightforward manipulation of money-power. It is no doubt a blessing that for the vast majority of us institutions such as male primogeniture no longer exist to poison family relations, but even so it seems to me that we vastly underestimate the psychological consequences of inheritable wealth for those who stand in line actually to inherit it. This does not of course constitute a widespread social problem, but it does throw into relief the way that power may be socially exerted and reflected in individuals' personal lives and relations. I cannot claim that my knowledge of people in this position is extensive, but it has struck me as interesting how often those I have come across – i.e. people who have wealthy parents and who profit or stand to profit by the relationship – seem simply to have failed to grow up. For such people as this, however advanced in years themselves, the parental shadow seems to fall heavily over them, in such a way that emotionally and socially they remain perpetual adolescents – angrily dependent, sulkily rebellious, rather unstable and changeable in their personal relations, apparently vocationally paralysed, i.e. dilettantish and unable to strike out for themselves in any independent direction. However firm our intentions, very few of us manage to be disinterested, and it is extremely difficult for even the most affectionate parent not to wield at least unconscious power over a son or daughter who stands to gain financially from the relationship. It is not the habit of psychologists to inquire closely into the financial background and circumstances of those whose 'behaviour' and 'attitudes' they are trying to understand. On the whole, I suspect, to do so would be far more enlightening than to pursue, for example, the much more common inquiries into sexual history.

Whatever the level of the socio-economic circumstances in which a given family finds itself – and I should stress that the above reflections constitute only the broadest and most impressionistic of sketches – none can escape the prevailing cultural climate, which rains equally on the just and the unjust, the advantaged and the disadvantaged. The setting in which emotionally deprived and economically oppressed men and women compete with each other for equal shares of satisfaction, the intrusion into personal relations of inequalities in economic power and its veiled abuse, the pursuit and inevitable frustration of the desire for 'understanding', all these lead almost necessarily to a state of affairs in which children's experience and perceptions are marshalled or distorted to satisfy parental ambitions or emotional alignments, to 'validate' familial mythology or to deny uncomfortable truths. If in this process the adults' power is not ruthlessly if unconsciously used to transmit forms of 'socialization' which are built, ultimately, on exploitation and violence, it is likely simply to be withdrawn as an available resource, in which case children merely grow up like weeds as their parents fend off any demand which intrudes on their search for personal satisfaction. This in fact does seem to be the ultimate destination of our individualistic pursuit of happiness – simple indifference to the fate of the next generation. It seems more and more to be the case that parents are coming to experience their children as a threat to their emotional peace and independence, as yet more competition for scarce satisfactions, so that adult power comes to serve the struggle for personal 'happiness' more than cultivation of a future for our progeny. This becomes the business of a professional stratum of educational and therapeutic 'experts'.

What seems increasingly to be characteristic of our 'relationships' as a whole is a lack of charity, an absence of the forbearance and respect in the face of 'otherness' which are necessary to an acceptance of each other as fully human. The perception of each other as vehicles of commodified satisfaction which market values impose feeds fantasied expectations, the inevitable frustration of which can only result in desperate neediness and anger. Human beings denied the possibility of acting *creatively* out into the world *for* something become in the end reduced to acting out dreams *destructively* in a way which pays no regard to the embodied actuality of their fellows. This tendency is clearly to be read in the often horrifyingly detached or fantastic sexual and aggressive preoccupations of modern literature and cinema, etc. ('enjoyment' of which necessitates a kind of defensive steeling of the sensibilities if one is not to emerge at least temporarily scarred) but is no less easily identified in the sense very many 'ordinary' people have these days of a pervasive *cruelty* in the world.

Frustration and neediness compounded by recognition of failure to meet the needs of others create a despair and *unintentional* cruelty (i.e. a form of cruelty carrying with it no sense of personal 'ownership') which are reflected as surely in our intimate relations as they are, for example, in the wider world of national and international affairs. The profoundly sinister, largely unseen but enormously complex apparatus of nuclear warfare, the South African policeman almost frenziedly whipping a peaceful demonstrator, and the father who regards with stony hatred the despair of a daughter he cannot love are not separate phenomena, but together speak to the way in which we have become caught up in issues of power and competition beyond our immediate comprehension or control. Any improvement in this state of affairs will depend on a great deal more than our merely 'working on our relationships'.

7

Growing Up and Taking Care

Understanding, as I have tried to show, does not equal cure. For the individual starting out on psychotherapy it often seems as if all that is needed for the relief of his or her nameless distress would be a clear sight of what the reasons for it are. But even though the gaining of such a clear sight may be a lengthy, painful and testing procedure, its difficulties are as nothing compared with those which arise once the mist disperses and the person can see quite clearly the nature of his or her predicament. For the predicament is where one *is*, and though one may be able to envisage in perfect detail where one would *like* to be, the greatest difficulties are encountered in knowing how to get there. There are, of course, some advantages in knowing where you are, and for many patients this is an improvement on the confusion and discomfort of their original condition, and indeed one which often they have to settle for, if only because their history or their situation precludes their being able to act on their world in such a way as significantly to change it. But even for those who do have some prospect of being able to influence their situation through their own conduct, the way is never less than daunting and always demands great effort and courage.

Precisely the same kind of constellation of difficulties, though on a vastly greater scale, faces the analysis, such as it is, presented in this book. Whatever clarity may have been gained through having broken free of the conceptual restraints placed on our understanding of human distress by the disciplinary structures, greedy individualism and meshed interests of a hierarchy of power, we are still no nearer to knowing how to change our lives or to escape the influences we may now see as damaging us. However, perhaps it is a little easier to catch a glimpse of how, if only we could change them, our lives *ought* to look: the ends may be fairly clear even if the means are as obscure as ever. In this chapter, then, I shall undertake the relatively uncomplicated task of suggesting what indications for less destructive and deluded ways of living seem to me to follow from the foregoing analysis. In the next, and final, chapter I shall discuss, without hoping to resolve, some of the difficulties and dilemmas involved in trying actually to bring into existence forms of social conduct which are, I think, easily enough identified as desirable.

For no particular reason other than convenience of organization, I shall divide into two broad strands this discussion of how, perhaps, our lives should be if we wish to escape the ravages of the pursuit of happiness. The first strand deals with our personal expectations of life and entails the necessity for growing up. The second deals with our relations with others and the world we live in, and entails the necessity for taking care. It is with some embarrassment that I find myself treading this territory, which is not customarily regarded as the legitimate habitat of 'scientific' psychologists, and I am afraid that what I write may sound too much like preaching. I do not, however, regard myself as in a different boat from anyone else, and though I certainly feel a degree of diffidence about this undertaking I make no apology for it: its justification will, I hope, be argued in the next chapter.

Growing Up

The blissful security of infancy – the inevitable if for some pitifully short foundation of our experience – is, as has been noted, not to be recaptured. In circumstances rather saner than those pertaining in the 'civilized' world towards the end of the twentieth century, it is likely to be the natural course of a person's life that it should, once delivered from the womb, turn progressively outwards towards the world. The process of growing up corresponds to the cultivation of a 'public' life in which the person is enabled, as well perhaps as obliged, to make a contribution to the social world before coming to the end of his or her brief sojourn in it. This is not to say that 'private' life – the internal world of feelings and 'relationships' – is unimportant or to be despised, but rather that it is of little interest to anyone other than the individual in question and those with whom he or she comes into intimate contact.

It is in the public sphere that one may have a more or less formal *function* through which one contributes to the world, and it is in the private sphere that one may tend to the concerns of the self. The 'pursuit of happiness' is properly a private matter, the *instrumental* use of one's body in a social context properly a public matter. We are, in ways and for reasons which may become a little clearer in the course of this discussion, chronically confused between the public and private spheres.

The possibility of public life confers a kind of dignity, a social as opposed to a purely personal value, even at the lowliest level. The doorman, for example, in his commissionaire's uniform, may for many be little more than a slightly comical symbol of petty authority, but the 'publicness' of his role at least permits him to wear an expression of pride which will almost certainly be absent from the face he watches in the bathroom mirror as he stands in his pyjamas cleaning his teeth. He contrasts strongly in this 'publicness' with the young girl who walks past him. His body, his privacy, is hidden behind his function, nobody's business but his own; her body is packaged and displayed as seductively as it can be made – she is imprisoned in a kind of cocoon of private sexuality which is at the same time constructed to be looked at. On the one hand her appearance issues the strongest invitation to desire, on the other she meets nobody's gaze, her eyes unseeing, her expression contemplating some secret inner space. Her determined avoidance of the gaze her objectified sexuality invites seems to acknowledge the inappropriateness of publicizing an essentially private concern. In any case, she is given no function but to be her body, a pure object; she has been turned inside-out.

The economic structures we inhabit rob most of us of any function extended out into public space, so that our existence becomes imploded into an impacted preoccupation with our selves and our needs; they *exploit* private impulse at the same time as *appropriating* public function.

But privacy is to be respected, not exploited. As far as there can be a 'point' to our lives, it must, surely, reside within the public sphere; to focus the point of living on the personal and perhaps idiosyncratic experiences of individuals and their particular satisfactions and gratifications is to give the private a degree of importance and centrality far beyond anything morally or rationally warrantable. Indeed, the emphasis on private satisfaction in our commercial culture is so inflated as to obscure the sphere of public living altogether. The promise of bliss holds us within an endless infancy, or at least makes it impossible for us to progress beyond a greedy adolescence, and in assuring us that this *is* the point of life, it in fact cruelly robs our lives of meaning. It is not merely that our longing for a blissful past beyond the reach of memory is nurtured and exploited, but it is also the case that in many ways the sphere of public living has contracted to a point where most people cannot enter it even if they want to. It may be true that in most 'developed' societies the world no longer imposes upon people a harsh necessity for growing up (our children are not forced to drop their toys so that they may lay their hands to the plough, indeed our adult lives are at least as engrossed with toys – mostly made in Japan – as is our childhood), but it is also true that if we wish to put away childish things we actually cannot find anything serious to do. In other words, growing up in our situation has ceased to be a natural process.

To observe that growing up is no longer a natural process is, however, not to imply that it is not a necessary one if we are to escape the disintegration and despair consequent upon meaning-lessness. We have, quite literally, bought the idea that the point of life is the pursuit of happiness, and so we have become, as it were, collapsed in on a life of private contemplation of how we feel. Private individualism of this kind leads to public (social) disintegration. It is far from the case that *really* life's 'problems' have been solved to the point where we can now just sit back and enjoy ourselves – even the most casual glance at the state of our own society, let alone of the rest of the world, reveals that this fantasy of the sixties no longer holds any plausibility at all. Furthermore, if ever that distant day should be reached when human society *does* seem to have solved all its problems, human beings will have to think of something better to do than just enjoy themselves having fun and therapy, for it does not take much imagination to see how deadening and futile such a life would be.

The greatest violence that is done to people in our society is to rob them of a public life. As people are persuaded by an unremitting barrage of commercial propaganda that their happiness lies in the indulgence and satisfaction of their private needs and impulses, they are simultaneously stripped of the possibility for developing and using talents, resources and interests which they can place at the disposal of others and enact for the public good. This is a large part of the reason for the despair which lies behind our satiation. Once again one is reminded of battery chickens, whose only difference from us lies, presumably, in their lack of a consciousness. Since it knows no other, the battery chicken (if only it could talk to itself) would no doubt believe that it existed in the best of all possible worlds, and would see the point of its existence as being fed regularly and nourishingly, kept in comfortable – if overcrowded – circumstances of even light and heat, and medicated to keep it free of disease and maintain its proper rate of growth. What the chicken would not see, of course, is that there is indeed an altogether darker and less bland purpose behind its pampered life of easy passivity, and even on the day of its sudden and terrifying end it would not realize what its life had been for. Our case is not so different, for our lives also have a purpose beyond that (the pursuit of happiness) which we can immediately see, and though it is one to which, if we are lucky, our private life is not sacrificed, it is certainly one which claims our public lives. It is however, for most of us, not a purpose of our own choosing nor one to which we would consider it right to subscribe, and for most of us also its nature is located at a point in the hierarchy of interest which we cannot even see. In order to develop our *own* purposes we need to break the unnatural barriers to our own maturity: if we do not grow up in response to the pressures of the world, we shall have to learn how to do so for ourselves.

The infrequency with which one comes across people who have achieved maturity is perhaps an indication of how difficult, in the modern world, it is to do so. Even from the perspective of purely private experience, to *grow* older, rather than simply to become advanced in years, is to leave an almost-memory of certain safety and blissful peace and to penetrate further and further into the uncertain and unknowable, to relinquish passivity for activity, to unwind oneself from wishful dreaming and in the process discover pains and sorrows which no mythology can eradicate. In order to embark upon any such risky journey, one needs a social world and a culture which at least make an effort to map the way as far as possible and to provide support at the most dangerous and distressing junctures. In fact, of course, that is precisely what is missing – at every hesitant step we are called back by seductive promises of security and ease and encouraged to regard any sign of departure from the standard aim of happy consumption as close to madnesss. Life does indeed tend to force the inevitable experiences of increasing age on those of us who live long enough, but our culture withholds from us (has repressed or failed to develop) both the conceptual equipment and the compassion we would need to make sense of what happens to us and perhaps to put it to some use in our public lives. Almost every milestone we pass – adolescent sexuality, marriage, parenthood, the departure of children, the demands of old age, death, to name but the most basic and obvious – is mystified by the apparatus of interest so that at any point we are likely to be stunned into guilty silence as we discover that our actual experience fails to match the social norms it pays to believe in, and at the first opportunity we are likely to fall back on comforting but illusory formulations which seem to relieve us of the necessity for progressing further into a threatening unknown.

This kind of process illustrates the meaning of the psychoanalytic term 'fixation'. We settle for that point of our development beyond which we dare not advance, and we elaborate a life out of the *safe* knowledge thus far gained. Sometimes the point settled for may not be very far along the chronological path at all – perhaps merely a matter of months. Unless as a society we provide people, as far as we are able, with both the understanding and the encouragement to risk and pass beyond the difficult and painful experiences which are bound to present themselves at intervals throughout their lives, we can scarcely be surprised when they settle for what they know best and baulk at entering areas of experience which lie, so to speak, outside their field of expertise.

We tend to traumatize our children early: rather than trying all we can to use our adult knowledge and power to stand in their position and to make sense *for* them of *their* experience, to make space in which they can act from their own perspective, we tend to impose upon them a cold objective gaze which monitors their every departure from our norms and enables us to force them back into the ways of *our* choosing. In this way, the child becomes terrified of its own 'interiority': it discovers that most of what it experiences and feels and thinks is not permissible, and so, as soon as it can, it opts for any state of 'objectivity' in which it seems to be moderately successful and reasonably comfortable, and beyond that state it does not pass.

Partly, this is because the exploitation of privacy for both commercial and disciplinary purposes, the spilling out of what is inside us into the field of view of others who need to sell us things as well as keep us under control, leads us vastly to over-estimate and over-extend the significance of our private lives and the way we feel inside ourselves. It is not that such feelings are unimportant – indeed, as I have indicated, they deserve the greatest respect and care – but rather that their importance does not extend so far as to account for or give meaning to our function as social beings. Once centred on how you *feel*, however, it becomes very difficult to concentrate unself-consciously on what you want to *do*, especially when what you feel seems to bear no relation to how you have been led to expect you *ought* to feel.

Most of us, I suspect, spend our lives elaborating a way of objective being discovered relatively early in life, rather than moving through a progression of subjective experience. The changing nature of one's embodied position in the world (given as much as anything by the alteration in one's circumstances) and the accretion of one's history which are necessarily consequent on becoming older, provide one with an endlessly unrolling sequence of experience which demands a capacity for continuously learning anew. For most of us, as already suggested, this is experienced rather as a series of incomprehensible blows to a (probably tacit) philosophy of life which we accepted early on as finished and immutable or else took over uncritically from the 'official' mythology of our time. Life is not seen as something 'open-ended' and new and requiring learning, but rather as a relatively fluid period of childhood followed by a relatively stable period of adulthood,* both calling for nothing more taxing than the acquisition of already clearly defined 'skills'. It is because of this sharp discrepancy

---

*An alternative to this conventional view is, however, put by Phillida Salmon in her *Living in Time*, Dent, 1985.

between the official mythology and what people actually experience of life and death and love and work that it is common for them to feel traumatized and to 'fixate' on what they know best. It is not difficult to think of examples – most of us know people who, whatever the situation they find themselves in, rather than *experiencing* it, work out within it their practised form of objectivity. The young man, for instance, who is always beautiful and clever no matter what is being asked of or enacted around him: his specialism in life is to be beautiful and clever, and his eyes are cast modestly down when he feels the eyes of others noting his beauty, and his aphoristic speech turns every occasion into an appreciation of his wit and intelligence. This kind of self-conscious objectivity is the curse of a society which penetrates private life with a public gaze, which maintains discipline and furthers interest by censoring our experience and so making it impossible for us to act out into public space without worrying too much how we look or feel. The result is that we become paralysed, unable to *function*. With a longing backward glance at a safer past we turn ourselves into pillars of salt.

In order to grow up, we have perhaps above all to learn renunciation rather than longing. All promises that we may return again to the blissful ease of infancy are false. Though we may entirely legitimately mourn its passing, and no doubt enjoy those beautiful if brief times when (as in falling in love) something like it seems to reappear, it is not wise to pine for the paradise which, because we cannot quite remember it, seems like a hope for the future. Wishful dreaming merely renders one vulnerable to commercial promises of its coming true and sucks one into a life in pursuit of the illusory. This is the entirely private life of personal satisfaction, which even if we could achieve 'fulfilment' would be totally devoid of meaning. The renunciation of bliss constitutes not some kind of self-imposed penance or unnecessary asceticism, but rather a sober recognition that a life lived in the public domain (i.e. one in which thought, feeling and action are turned outward to the world) is one which necessarily involves difficulty, uncertainty, isolation and a measure of pain.

What is needed is a degree of stoicism. What so often we anticipate as unbearable we might better come to see as inevitable, and possibly even not all that bad. (The aim here of course is not to submit stoically to the authority or values of an immutable hierarchy of power, but to liberate oneself from the mythology through which it furthers its interests and maintains its discipline.) There is, certainly, not such virtue in emotional pain that one need seek it out, but there is an inevitability about it which makes repression of any familiarity with it counterproductive: no life spent running away from the inevitable can be particularly worth while. There *are* risks inherent both in forming attachments to others and in trying to make whatever contribution one can to the public good, but a knowledge of risk and a readiness to experience loss, rejection or failure actually make them easier to bear when they do occur than does the single-minded pursuit of gratification.

There is, of course, nothing the matter with the enjoyment of private pleasure or happiness (nor with eccentric personal suffering) but, being private, they need to be covered by a decent reticence. It is characteristic of modern marketing strategy to drag values and feelings out of the private domain and to harness their power as 'motivators' to saleable commodities. In this way the domain of public life – the sphere of conduct in which we act outwardly to and with each other *for* something beyond our private satisfaction – has become inverted into a kind of public privacy, i.e. emptied of public significance and filled instead with objectified personal feelings and needs. Our privacy and interiority have been invaded, raped, and dragged out for public scrutiny in a way which only seems without shame because we are *all* involved. The barriers by means of which a personal interiority used to be defended, and which thus permitted the living of a private life, have one by one been broken down, and our legitimate concern with ourselves and our feelings has been exposed to an objective gaze and made public property. One thinks, for example, of the erosion of the right to the dignity of a surname through the generalized use of first names by which was once conferred a gift of intimacy. The touching and gazing and exteriorizing of thoughts and feelings which are the stock-in-trade of the therapy industries are little more than techniques for making us less resistant to the demands and blandishments of the market as well as more uniformly vulnerable and obedient to the discipline of social norms. All this, it seems, amounts to another form of one-dimensionality: in becoming fused into a single realm of publicly private commodification, our lives have lost both a decent and enjoyable (or sufferable) privacy as well as the possibility for altruistic action in a public domain.

It is not, then, that our private lives are unimportant or of no consequence, nor that the pleasures and pains they contain should be a matter of indifference to us, but that they are indeed a private concern. We need to *take back* our private lives, to retrieve them from the intrusive interests both of the market and of social discipline (norms) so that we can live them, in privacy, as diversely, eccentrically, and if the occasion demands as unhappily as we like. It is indeed a particular privilege of the grown-up to live a private life however he or she likes. (It is, furthermore, the business of the psychotherapist, if asked, as far as possible to help people to do precisely that, and not to try to push them into conformity with some standardized conception of 'mental health'. Rather than being, as they unwittingly too often are, representatives of a form of social discipline, psychotherapists could better become the reticent and unheroic assistants of people whose private struggles are nobody's business but their own and that of those in whom they choose to confide. In this way psychotherapists should occupy a status position more similar to that of those old-fashioned physicians who in order to test their patients' urine had to taste it than to that of magicians or social engineers; there is, in other words, not a great deal of glamour or mystery in examining the difficulties and distress we encounter in our private lives.)

While an individual's happiness or despair may indeed reside in his or her private life, the *point* of living has more relevance to the public sphere. Indeed, the very possibility of being able to contribute to the society in which one lives may well redeem or give meaning to a life lived otherwise in misery. Even were our exclusive interest in people's private lives compassionate rather than commercial, we should still, by draining off the possibility for public conduct, render them meaningless. Suffering is not to be desired for itself, but better suffering with the possibility of redemption than a purely private bliss.

It is almost impossible to envisage what sort of society it would be which permitted or encouraged all its members to turn their lives towards some public function. Our own society, certainly, is diametrically opposed to this: it siphons off the possibility of 'other-directed' (altruistic) conduct in order to commodify its products and sell them back to people as consumers. But if there is any 'point' to living, it must surely lie in what we can do; our embodied organisms are surely *for* something other than their own satisfaction. Only if we live in the perpetual 'now' of the advertiser's euphoric world could we really believe that a life which is not permitted to develop and apply its talents for the benefit of all is not, no matter how great its private satisfaction, a life wasted. It is the instrumentality of the body which renders it indispensable to the evolution of a social world, not its capacity for enjoyment, nor even, I would suggest, its inclination towards spiritual 'fulfilment'.

It is indeed the very uni-dimensionality of our materialistic philosophy which leads us to think it essential that we should know what the 'point' of living is in any case. We tend to assume, for example, that unless we can identify a 'point', life becomes point*less* or absurd. But there is no compelling reason to believe that, for there to be a point, we should know what it is. It is, after all, likely to take many more thousands of centuries before we have got as far as learning how decently to live together, without worrying about what the point of it all might be. The very most we can hope to do is make what contribution we can in the vanishingly brief time available to us. In view of the heartless waste of talent, the systematic destruction of intelligence and the commercialized emptying-out of mentality which, in particular, characterize our treatment of the young, it seems to me that to aim at maximizing the possibility of our contributing, through our embodied instrumentality, to a future none of us can foretell, is far from an unworthy or uninspiring goal.

For it is certainly not that there is nothing for us to do. A world which is built on injustice, inequality and violence, in which the relative comfort and 'happiness' of a few is founded on the exploitation and degradation of the vast majority, leaves plenty of room for improvement, and we certainly need not yet despair that human life is rendered meaningless through its very affluence and technological success (in this respect it is interesting again to remember that all those epochs of our history which have been characterized by self-confident assertions of comfort and sufficiency in fact seem to have derived their security from a basis in some form of slavery). Far from there being 'nothing to do' the domain of public life is in fact empty behind the illusion of activity created by the pervasive concern with what is in truth private indulgence (the moral bankruptcy of Western politics may perhaps be seen as testimony to this state of affairs: politicians become the cautious representatives or 'front' men and women for the interests of managerial, marketing and military power, and public policy is sacrificed to and for private interest).

It is a frequent complaint of 'patients' growing out of their longing for the bliss of infancy that their struggle to influence the circumstances of their lives 'doesn't have any effect'. This, again, seems to rest on the failure of a mature appreciation of scale: somehow, it seems, we have come to accept the values of instancy (instant availability and instant success) to the point where we lose sight of the smallness and relative insignificance of the individual. We have bought the belief that if one cannot change the world it is not worth trying, and so we become morally and politically paralysed. Part of the process of growing up entails the recognition that 'trying' is something to be done whether or not it has any degree of observable success. We have to reckon with the wastefulness of human society, to accept what is a fact *as* a fact: not only is it in most cases impossible to tell whether one's efforts in a given direction are or have been of any avail, but one must be prepared for the near certainty that they will have no *measurable* effect at all. Societies evolve through the agency of their members, but with a profoundly disheartening degree of redundancy – for every contribution that 'succeeds' there will be countless contributions which, at the very least, appear to go unnoticed. This state of affairs is an occasion for neither complacency nor despair, but sober recognition of it will at least militate against a belief in magic which can in the end only weaken our purchase upon our predicament.

Both the future of the species and the meaning of the individual's life cannot but be attended by great uncertainty. Despite the confident promise of the 'experts' to reveal and train us in the 'skills' required, there are no guarantees concerning the course of our lives, if only because that depends as much upon the context in which they occur as on the personal aims we have. The conduct of a life cannot be reduced to a technical performance of achievement or acquisition, but opens out into a range of possibilities which can only be acted *into* with faith. Faith is thus not a wishy-washy substitute for technical certainty, a form taken by lack of knowledge, but rather a necessary attitude or stance without which life cannot be lived except as private self-indulgence. Faith, moreover, does not have to be faith *in* anything more than possibilities which one cannot see, meanings not yet revealed, values whose worth one will never have a chance to measure.

Taking Care

It is not easy to think of the privileges and obligations of growing up in any terms other than those relating to an economics of consumption, the values of which are essentially passive and mechanically automatic. Thus progressive maturity becomes a question of the widening availability of certain commodities or pleasures (initiation into smoking, drinking, sex and 'adult' entertainment, availability of credit facilities, mortgages, etc.) and responsibility in observing certain legal and fiscal rules (e.g. in relation to taxation, military obligations, etc.). Since our ethics are those of the market-place and our view of knowledge and learning mechanistic and 'objective', we tend not to regard the transmission of our culture as a central task of all those 'embodied organisms' who go to make up our society, but rather as something which can safely be, and probably should be, left to professional experts of one kind or another. The rest of us can then get on with the serious business of making enough money to enjoy ourselves.

If, however, one takes seriously the argument put forward earlier in this book that indeed we *are* embodied organisms, that we are formed in the context of a history and a current set of circumstances whose effects are likely to be ineradicable, and that the society we build is the creation of human agency rather than the result of some kind of inexorable, natural objectivity, then it begins to become evident that one of the greatest responsibilities of maturity resides in the fact that we ourselves are the custodians and transmitters of our culture. What is known about the world of human society, and what therefore forms the basis of its further evolution (or indeed dissolution), is passed on to later generations *through* us: our culture is transmitted and developed through its assimilation and elaboration in the embodied practice of people. We cannot, then, merely pursue happiness while leaving the stewardship of the social world to nameless experts without risking a fundamental rupture in our cultural evolution and the complete loss of any sense of meaning to our lives.

It is, for example, easy to see how human knowledge and craft can be wiped out in two or three decades if it does not travel *through people* from one generation to the next. Even though the invention of printing 'de-skilled' large sections of the population by removing from them the necessity for the 'organic' transmission of knowledge, at least that knowledge is to some extent recoverable (if only with great effort) from books. In the case of mechanized knowledge, however, not only do we risk losing sight of the origins of our knowledge altogether (human knowledge literally *disappears into* the computer program in such a way that it is not recoverable without the aid of complex machines the destruction or non-comprehension of which would necessitate the re-invention of the knowledge) but we also render people functionless, and it is above all this which creates despair. It seems to me to follow from this that it is an essential part of human, and particularly of adult, existence to pay respect to our own nature as organisms and the organic nature of our culture by taking care both of each other and of those structures and institutions of the man-made social and cultural world which we wish to preserve and develop. This means taking care *of* people as ends in themselves and taking care *that* the best possible conditions are created for the performance of their functions (i.e. that we value people's instrumentality above their economic worth as consumers).

Attention to the conditions which make possible a public life would do much to alleviate what so many of us experience as purely private pain. The manipulation of people as units of consumption and re-recordable registers of fashion (in cultural as well as material life) places them in an endless, self-indulging present which has no past (in the sense of organic tradition) and no future (in the sense of evolving purpose). Rather than trying to 'normalize' the infinite range of differences between people and to 'pathologize' the extraordinary tenacity with which they live out their experience, we should be attending to those very conditions which make culture historically transmissible and the future open to forms of social evolution which cannot now even be guessed at. We should, in other words, seek to nurture, not reduce, the diversity and tenacity with which cultural forms are embodied in people. For older generations to attempt to shape younger ones to predetermined ends and ideas concerning the 'good life' amounts no matter how good their intentions to a form of spiritual murder, since by this means the young are deprived of the one function (to open up a future) which may give life a sense of meaning. But most of our effort seems to be put into repressing or destroying those very factors which make it possible to develop one's gifts to the full and to become unself-consciously absorbed in public activity.

As already suggested, mechanistic ways of thinking about human experience and learning threaten to lead to a catastrophic loss of social as well as practical and intellectual ability in both range and depth. Precisely because of the organic nature of human experience one cannot quickly replace what has been lost to human mentality, although, by neglecting to pay attention to the importance of history and embodiment, one can very quickly wipe out human culture. Ivan Illich* writes of having seen children of ten in New York slums who 'could not speak a word, although the television was blaring, sometimes two televisions in the same welfare apartment'. Novels such as *Last Exit to Brooklyn* should have alerted us years ago to the likely fate of a society which ignores 'organic' values. Despair and brutality are the entirely natural recourse of people who have been dislocated from the flow of human culture and deprived of the possibility of putting their bodies to good use. It is scarcely surprising that both our 'entertainment' and our 'news' media should be almost obsessively concerned with rape and murder, since these are the rational end-points of any disintegrated society which is concerned more or less solely with removing the obstacles to getting what you want. Very pertinently does R. D. Laing write that all of us are born as Stone Age babies (though even Stone Age babies were born into a culture which was transmitted through embodied human beings).

One does not have to search our own inner cities very far before coming across indications of what an uncultivated Stone Age baby may become in this 'technologically advanced' society. Four boys, for example, idle down a back street in the city centre, truanting from school one week-day morning. Every few yards they stop, for no apparent purpose, looking around them with a kind of

*Vernacular values, in Satish Kumar (ed.), *The Schumacher Lectures*, Abacus, 1982.

menacing casualness, aimless and yet embodying some kind of want. One of them gobs every twenty seconds or so with a contemptuous accuracy, exercising listless pride in a negative art. Their faces have an expression of sardonic brutality, a youthful energy but empty of purpose and unlit by intelligence; their eyes are watchful, but veiled, unfocused and dead. They seem sadly at home in this quiet, unpeopled street with its few tradesmen's shops, service entrances to the backs of stores, empty Coca-Cola tins and refuse blown from black polythene sacks; there are no demands here that they cannot meet. The overwhelming impression is that these are wasted people, bodies in which no function dwells. They seem to exist outside of any developed culture, unanimated by any refined tradition, and there is about them a heavily threatening air – one senses that they do not know how to do anything but respond to their own most basic, private impulses, that they could not negotiate social rituals which have become to them mysteries bristling with the risk of ridicule; one senses that they could only take.

A number of social phenomena – for example the strange mixture of therapy and programming, the gradual fusion of teaching with social work, the transformation of 'parenting skills' into a professional training 'package' to be delivered by experts – suggest that we have become extremely confused over the means as well as the ends of taking care of those for whom we are responsible. The ineradicability of human experience coupled with the ample evidence we have of its so-frequently distressing nature should make us much more concerned about what we want to teach our children and why, and far less sanguine about being able to control or alter the 'input' in any way we happen to feel like. Confidence in technology makes us scornful of tradition, and it may no doubt be true that sentimental attachment to tradition for its own sake can have a deadening effect on cultural evolution. However, recognition that a culture can be stably transmitted only through the painstaking induction of 'Stone Age babies' into a *history* is something that should make us revise our too-unthinking trust in 'techniques' of training and therapy. What actually happens to people is of the most fundamental importance, and the nature of the world in which they are located will have far more significance for their experience than will the latest fashions in educational 'technique'.

At the very simplest level, our faith in and dependence upon 'experts' leads many people (both parents and teachers) to overlook the importance of *doing things with* children, of passing on to them what we know through living, embodied contact, just as it was passed on to us. Nobody entirely in his or her right mind would expect someone to learn to play the violin purely from audio-visual displays, and yet there is no difference in principle between the ways in which this and more simple kinds of knowledge are learned. Even where there is anything to be learned beyond the means of mere private gratification, because our own functional activities have become so minutely specialized, managerially fractured, pressured by time, and often simply meaningless, children tend not to be admitted into a participatory involvement in the lives of those adults to whom they are closest. Children occupy a separate world, or rather a separate market in which they consume commodities designed specifically for them (e.g. 'toys') rather than starting to practise functions mastery of which would admit them in due course to an adult world. This has the result that knowledge and ability die out with the bodies of an older generation by which they have been organically acquired, while the bodies of the younger generation are for the most part empty of instrumental function. Even when a talented boy or girl teaches him- or herself something (say, for example, playing the guitar) by virtue of persistent curiosity and observation, the result, even if greatly admired and commercially successful, often betrays a kind of untutored rawness, an uncultivated creative potentiality which, however, would need the knowledge and tradition of a culture were it to be fully realized. The rhetoric of our marketing society betrays well enough an awareness of this kind of loss – in prattling of 'excellence', for example, it somehow hopes to compensate for its systematic destruction. We end up with a culture in which each generation discovers for itself anew forms of unrefined knowledge the 'excellence' of which is never honed beyond the span of an individual life: yet another form of 'built-in obsolescence'.

If we need to pay much closer attention to the *way* people learn, we may well need to be far less controlling than we are about *what* they learn. Only a society interested in establishing a disciplined conformity will try to legislate for exactly what experience a person ought to have, and I do not wish to suggest that we need to construct any *particular* kind of world for our children. The very openness of the future means that the wider and more exuberant the diversity of their knowledge, interests and talents, the better. What *is* important to remember is that whatever world people do find themselves in, they learn its lessons well, and we do therefore need to consider very carefully what we want our own contribution to it to be. We have in fact not developed anything like an articulate understanding of what the *forms* of 'taking care' might be. We are much more tempted, in accordance with the values of technology, to develop ideas about the *content* we consider desirable for programmes of instruction, etc., and in that very process have substituted a mythology of training for a philosophy of learning.

There is, of course, an enormous amount of inarticulate knowledge about teaching and learning embodied in all kinds of people who have care of others at all levels of society, whether informally or formally, privately or institutionally, but when such people do try to articulate their knowledge they usually do so in the prescribed technological manner with which we are so familiar, and while this does not necessarily invalidate their actual conduct, it certainly does not facilitate it. I know many people – parents as well as professional 'carers' – who in fact develop and cultivate with the greatest sensitivity and intelligence a world in which their charges can grow, who teach and transmit an embodied mentality and a cultural ethics of the highest complexity, without having the slightest *articulate* idea of what they are doing. If asked, they are as likely as not to fall back on the crassest banalities drawn from current 'skills' or 'relationship' jargon. Not the least penalty of our mechanistic, ahistorical, individualizing and objectifying culture is that it deprives us of a language in which we can elaborate what we know (and by means of which also, of course – and hence the deprivation – we could begin conceptually to dismantle the ideology which underpins our way of life).

Loving cultivation of a child's interests and abilities, painstaking construction of a world in which he or she may practise them, respect for the embodied experience through which traditional knowledge is communicated – all those ways in which care is *actually* taken form no part of our official systems of training and treatment. This is of course not to suggest that they could or should be formalized into a system of technical expertise, in which they would swiftly be appropriated by 'professionals', but rather to suggest that we should value and where possible facilitate their very informality. It would help in this to recognize our formal systems of 'care' for what they are (i.e. institutions built around a disciplinary interest) and to try to develop a language by means of which we could talk to each other in terms which are, precisely, subjective and informal (i.e. as nearly as possible uncorrupted by power).

One cannot, of course, say how this might be achieved. One thing, certainly, would be to withdraw from the 'experts' the right tacitly accorded them to have the final (and indeed often the only) say in how things should be done. Because we have come to see knowledge and learning as purely technical matters we have not only become blind to the manner of their transmission, but indifferent to the structures in which they are organically embedded. Traditions associated with human intercourse of all kinds, whether in work, 'gendered' activity, religious ritual and so on, are likely to be seen as unintelligible or absurd merely because there issues from them no digitally unambiguous 'read-out' of their meaning. The wisdom built into the apprenticeship model of learning (and not only, of course, in the manual trades), the knowledge of social and familial roles and conduct transmitted through direct participation in them, the understanding that ability is acquired only through the taking of pains (and is then not quickly forgotten) — all these ways of coming to know have become atrophied or lost because they have to be passed on through a process of embodied activity rather than articulated in verbal instructions, and since we overvalue the latter we cease to practise the former.

Our preference for professionally specifiable, highly symbolized and mechanizable 'knowledge' is simply a mistake, and one which empties out an impoverished culture into machines while rendering us blind to what we do learn from the world. Children know television advertising jingles and the detailed personal histories of popular singers and guitar players; they learn informally from the culture which engages their interest, but because we *define* learning in terms of the highly oversimplified 'modules' of school curricula, we barely even notice what is indelibly finding its way into the structure of their bodies. We no longer initiate them into the social processes of a communal life not only because these are in any case sadly deprived of meaning, but also because we assume that when necessary they will be able to get all they need to know from audio-visual displays put on by the experts.

It may be the case that no society has yet been very good at articulating and understanding the processes whereby it evolves, and hence at preserving those traditional forms within which its members' conduct may carry its culture forward. Part of the reason for the rejection and abandonment of traditional modes of cultural transmission may be that the, so to speak, embodied rituals through which they were enacted tended to be accompanied by a justificatory rhetoric which lost authority through its very implausibility. The ethics of Christian society, for example, are unquestionably weakened for most people when associated with an insistence on a belief in miracles, immaculate conception, resurrection, etc., which can no longer command credence. But as long as the culture was embodied in the traditional practices of its members the rhetoric never really mattered. A problem with modern society is that *we really do believe* in our techno-scientific rhetoric to the point where we have almost ceased to pay attention to anything but words and images, and our actual embodied existence has slid out of sight to become the prey of repressed interest and hence the unidentified source of our distress.

We need to recover our knowledge of the world and of the conditions of human experience and learning in terms of an informal language which strives after truth rather than authority, compassion rather than power, care rather than control (a language, in fact, which reflects what Ivan Illich calls 'vernacular' rather than market values). No society, as far as I am aware, has yet tried in any concerted or protracted way to develop such an 'ideology', though there have of course always been scattered individuals who have argued for it; perhaps all this shows is that there are little grounds for optimism about the future.

Knowledge of the essential conditions for the development of an embodied existence capable of contributing to public life is automatically repressed by the *dis*embodied technical language of training and therapy, which on the contrary moulds people to disciplinary norms and shapes them as the means to commercially determined ends. The modern conception of an ideally adjusted social being, technically programmed for maximum success and happiness, sets up an entirely fictional standard which everyone fails more or less painfully to meet. The practical effect of this is to engender in people a guilty awareness of their own shortcomings in relation to the norms even while they insist that those with whom they 'have relationships' should themselves strive harder to reach them. We have, in short, a pervasive sense that we are not as we should be. If, however, we could begin to see ourselves and each other as embodiments of ineradicable experience and, because of this, as bearers of a multifarious knowledge of the world which has contributions to make to a future we cannot predict, we might then learn to 'relate to' each other more as what we are rather than as what we think we ought to be, and to treat each other as ends rather than as means.

When reading, for example (but perhaps also especially), the works of Dickens, one gets a feeling of entering a strangely unfamiliar world in which others exist as distinct entities with a value inseparable from their individuality, as living forces to be attended to and learned from because of rather than in spite of their 'otherness'. There is something in the brilliance of Dickens's caricatures which draws *sympathetic* attention to the way a person is made in relation to a context rather than a standard; though he disapproves of and frequently punishes his villains, there is nevertheless behind their villainy the sense of a history which cannot be wished away, and those characters he approves of are appreciated because of their very quirkiness. This feels more like a forgotten than a fictional world, but in any case points to a way of seeing and treating people which has become almost foreign to us. Our instinct is to approve of those people who most completely meet our standards for the gratification of our needs, and we do not on the whole see it as the task of 'relationship' literally to *learn* to live with the idiosyncrasies of the other. And yet, if it really is the case that we are each of us inescapably the unique embodiment of a particular history, the 'Dickensian' approach to 'otherness' is by far the more appropriate, if also more demanding.

Because, inevitably, there will be areas of your experience which do not overlap with mine, things you know about, as part as your emotional embodiment, of which I have no inkling, and because similarly my experience is shaped by events of which you have no knowledge or understanding, we must both take care not to confuse each other with our dreams of who we are and ought to be. Perverted by the blandishments of a commercial culture which markets people, we expect to be able to transform ourselves within relationships in such a way as to meet each other's needs, and if we cannot we assume that it must be because of a lack, if not of willingness, at least of 'interpersonal skills' or sexual 'technique', and so on. If the person does not come up to the demands of 'the relationship' he or she must either be trained to 'shape up' or exchanged for someone more malleable. You must fit my dreams, and I yours.

But it is part of the process of growing up to realize that some dreams are just dreams and will not be fulfilled, and it is part of a process whereby we might take care of each other to learn to accord to each other a reality which can be neither changed nor penetrated – the aim of 'relationship' cannot therefore be 'understanding'. My guess is that people who vow that their 'long-term relationship' shall be for better or for worse do so more as an expression of an exalted passion in the present than out of a sober commitment to a future in which the balance between better and worse may really be judged as no better than even. If we expect our 'relationships' to be matters of more or less unalloyed satisfaction we are certain to discover that they will be for worse rather than for better, but if we could learn to appreciate and protect each other's difference without having to 'understand' it, to tolerate and perhaps even be ready to explore a degree of isolation, we might then be able to avoid inflicting upon each other some of the pain we currently take as justified in our pursuit of happiness.

In renouncing the standards we set for each other we would allow ourselves to emerge before each other as embodied presences each containing a core of private 'interiority' which we would feel no compulsion to reveal even if we could. Rather than being the transparent vehicles of 'relationship', trembling with anxiety before the discipline of the norm and pierced by the gaze of a market searching for deficits to be made good, we might become people whose privacy, beyond the point at which it could be shared in a privileged intimacy, would be appreciated, protected or cherished, not emptied out into an arena where it becomes the focus of competition or frustrated rage.

On the 19 June 1896, Tolstoy* noted what seemed to him a 'very important' thought: 'What is beauty? Beauty is what we love. *I don't love him because he's beautiful, but he's beautiful because I love him.*' In other words, it is in the commitment to the other (for example in coming to know the other's difference) that the value of 'relationship' lies, not in the acquisition *through* the relationship of commodity-characteristics which the other possesses somehow objectively.

Only very partially can we repair after the event the damage we so easily inflict upon each other in the pursuit of happiness. It is for this reason above all that we need to establish now procedures of care-taking which will bear fruit only in a future we shall not see. Our most reliable guide in the formulation of our conduct in this respect is not the longing for an unattainable bliss but rather the private knowledge of pain. For though the knowledge is private, the pain is not merely personal, but arises from an embodiment in the world which is our common fate. It is not only you who are the victim of the other's indifference, contempt or spite, but the other is the victim of yours: you are other for others exactly as much as they are other for you. This is a fact which is necessarily overlooked in the struggle for resources which the pursuit of happiness entails; the inevitable individualism of the latter reduces universality to, at most, a grudging reciprocity, and transforms the public world into a projection of private dreams in which others become sacrificed to the needs of an insatiable 'self' or its various extensions (family, tribe, nation, 'the free world', etc.). It is the sensations of our bodies which give us knowledge of the world we share: as close as we can ever get to it, reality is revealed most undeniably in the experience of pain. One might almost say that reality is rooted in pain, and over and over again it is the pure sensation of pain which calls us back from disembodied reverie to habitation of a common world. And it is only in the knowledge that your embodiedness exposes you to the same risks as mine that we may make common cause to share the world. Lust for power and fantasies of invulnerability, trust in the magic of technical cure, lead us only into dreams of destruction.

The only way significantly to reduce the virtually universal distress and damage which our way of life causes is to construct social institutions which take account of the 'organic embodied-

Tolstoy's Diaries, vol. 2, op. cit.

ness' of our experience, the way we learn, etc., and to replace the 'pursuit of happiness' with an ethical awareness capable of making room for generosity, love, justice, equality and truth (i.e. values which – it cannot be overstressed – are *necessarily* sacrificed in a way of life which depends on competition and the creation of illusion). There will no doubt always be a place for therapy (i.e. for kindness, encouragement and comfort), but it is surely too much to expect a professionalized, and hence interest-saturated, therapy industry somehow to replace or take over the function of an ethics of human conduct.

However, although the statement of what needs to be done is so obvious as to be almost embarrassingly trite, one is still no nearer being able to see how to do it. The difficulties, certainly, seem insuperable, and it is virtually impossible for us even to imagine how we could find the courage to renounce our current ways of doing things, if only because we are all equally restrained by the enticing safety of familiarity from venturing into forms of conduct of which we have no practised understanding. Not that a reorientation of our lives, just supposing that we could make it, would necessarily be all gloom and self-sacrifice. The renunciation of a commodified gratification which is in any case illusory and the readiness to inhabit a degree of private isolation which is in any case inevitable may not be asking as much as it at first sight appears. Just as 'patients' who do screw up their courage to launch themselves into situations previously imagined as impossibly terrifying often find the reality positively liberating, so escape from the discipline of the norm, if only we could effect it, might prove to be a joyous relief. But this cannot be a 'boot-strap' operation to be achieved through exhortation or will power. Our conduct and our way of life are held in place by that world to which they are a rational response (in the sense elaborated in Chapter 4), and we are the embodied products of a history from which there is no escape.

The present – our current predicament – is, I suspect, irredeemable to an extent far beyond anything our self-deceiving therapeutic optimism has permitted us to see, and indeed there seems to be little sign that we are going to employ anything more substantial than 'public relations' and the machinery of illusion to appear to counter a continued squandering of human (not to mention other) resources. The damage we have done, and the damage we do now, will be felt for generations. If the future is to be rescued, it will not be through magic or wishful thinking, but through the creation of a social structure which encourages us to take care of each other.

8

Morality and Moralism

It is hard to conceive of a society in which all its members actually treat each other well. Presumably there has never been one. There have been, and are, societies in which a (usually religious) ethical code prescribes how people ought to treat each other even though they fail lamentably to live up to it. It is becoming increasingly apparent that contemporary Western society has no such ethical code. The empty shell of a system of Christian ethics, having for many centuries been laid siege to by the interests of power, has at last been taken over by the values of the market: Christianity becomes simply another way of getting things, achieving 'fulfil-ment' or a kind of exclusive 'salvation'. Most of us, therefore, live in a society in which there is no formal moral authority, no ethically based, publicly institutionalized code of conduct to which people subscribe in common. This is not to say, of course, that people do not still behave decently towards one another, but the grounds of this decency are hidden away tacitly and informally (and vulner-ably) in their private lives. The maxims of public life centre around competition, cost-effectiveness and the 'creation of wealth'. Ours, in short, is no longer an ethical community.

There are many perfectly understandable reasons for this state of affairs, but I suspect that the most important are those of which 'ordinary people' are least aware. For many people moral attitudes and prescriptions have too often been associated either with no longer credible religious magic or with hypocritical abuse of auth-ority for them to be able to submit to rules which so often turn out to be in somebody else's interest. The gradual fusion since mediaeval times of religious ethics with powerful commercial inter-ests has more recently accelerated to culminate in the supplantation of the former by the latter, has rendered moral understanding increasingly obscure, and has bred an entirely justifiable distrust of what has come to be seen as moralism. However, by far the most important reason for the disappearance of what one might call a 'public ethical code' is that its continuation would place unacceptable restraints on commercial exploitation. However brutal the mediaeval feudal lords may have been, and however corrupt the Church, at least, officially, they were not supposed to be. We have now reached a stage when the precepts of exploitation and self-interest are being slid into the place of moral values which can scarcely any longer be remembered.

The very idea of 'morality' – again understandably – is likely to arouse in people a range of unfavourable reactions. Apart from those who feel confident that they know what 'moral standards' are and are only too ready to say who ought to be made to conform to them, most people are quite likely to feel embarrassed, suspicious or contemptuous if asked explicitly to define what moral conduct in the public sphere might be. Morality has in this way come to be associated with sentimentality, hypocrisy, or 'unscientificness'.

However, unless morality is rescued from its obscurity – what is even almost a state of ignominy – and reinstated at the centre of our public life, it is hard to see how we can begin to construct a society worth living in. There are some ways, obviously, in which this will not happen. For example, morality as the revelation of a magical religious authority is surely something no longer likely to command widespread acceptance (far more likely, perhaps, is a resurgence of moral consciousness as the result of some kind of global catastrophe). Rather than having ethical standards imposed upon us through either magic or the law, it may be that we have reached a stage where, if we are to survive socially, we shall have in some way willingly to adopt an ethics of public life as our own. To employ an analogy which I have no doubt is dubious from many points of view, it is as if, having overthrown parental authority (religious morality) and 'enjoyed' a prolonged and irresponsible adolescence (the pursuit of happiness) we must now take upon ourselves the cares and responsibilities of adulthood and create out of our own ethical awareness and conduct a world in which human society can continue to evolve. Whether we can actually do this must seem doubtful if only because it is impossible to see what changes in our circumstances will force such a course upon us. It can certainly do no harm, however, to try to clarify what might be meant by 'moral' conduct.

It is important at the outset to distinguish 'morality' from 'moralism'. The form in which the majority of us these days are most likely to encounter overt discussion or prescription of 'moral values' is perhaps as pronouncements by one individual or group concerning what other individuals or groups ought to do or how they ought to conduct themselves. Thus, it seems to me, it is characteristic of moralistic injunctions that they are one-sided, and most frequently they are delivered by the stronger or more privileged as admonishments to the weaker or less privileged concerning how they should behave. Moralism is thus usually designed to protect the interests or 'image' of the relatively more powerful in their efforts to maintain others in their position of relatively less power. The idea, for example, that those who are well off in our society owe their fortune to some kind of *moral* superiority is taken as an entitlement for them to lecture the less fortunate in the ways of prudence and thrift, when they might better consider the purely logical dependence of wealth upon poverty and the social issues raised thereby.

Moralism is typically exemplified in the imputations of blame through which, as was argued in Chapter 4, the inequalities and injustices of our society are 'explained' as the moral failings of individuals. It is characteristic of moralism to attempt to cast morality in an explanatory form, either as causes of distress or failure or as motives which may be appealed to in exhortations to bear with adversity. But, of course, moral precepts are not things or forces which can be appealed to as operating somehow mechanically inside people, but rather are formulated as guides to public conduct. People, clearly, may conduct themselves morally or immorally, but they do not do things *because of* morality or immorality.

Moralism 'privatizes' morality. 'Moral responsibility', writes the archpriest of monetarism,* 'is an individual matter, not a social matter.' This, of course, leaves one conveniently placed to chide individuals who have succumbed to misfortune for their lack of moral fibre while allowing public conduct to be determined by the dictates of 'the market'. The 'invisible hand' of the market relieves one of the disagreeable necessity for deciding whether one's public activity is right or wrong, since its guidance is regarded as somehow infallible. Moral values thus become prescriptions identifiable by powerful people whose public conduct is seen itself as somehow above moral judgment, and applied to private individuals usually in the form of explanations concerning the personal failings that have led to their lack of success. The apparatus of interest, by transforming morality into moralism, turns it to its own advantage: the undoubted force of moral precept is deflected from its valid function of guiding public conduct and reshaped as a mystifying 'explanation' (as individual fault) of evils which are in fact the consequence of an immoral abuse of power.

One of the most striking and interesting things about the concept of morality itself is precisely its force. However disguised its operation or mystified its application, morality will simply not go away. Despite a widespread dissatisfaction people seem to feel with having to base their conduct on anything so vague and uncertain as moral judgment, and despite also the success of technological approaches which are based on a science supposedly 'value free', we can still, it seems, not dispense with words like 'right' and 'good' and 'ought'. It is no doubt easy to confuse technical with moral prescription: there are many areas in which accurate knowl-

*M. Friedman, *Free to Choose*, Penguin Books, 1980.

edge of how to do something has replaced the necessity for argument over which approach might be 'right' or 'wrong'. But to conclude from this that technical 'know-how' reduces the need for moral judgment is based on an obvious confusion between 'right' and 'wrong' in their moral sense and their use in the sense of 'effective' and 'ineffective'. The passion to be free of moral uncertainty results over and over again in attempts to find infallible guidelines which will remove from us the necessity for thinking about whether or not we *ought* to do something. Despite conclusive philosophical arguments that one can never replace an 'ought' with an 'is' – i.e. never decide what it would be right to do merely through a knowledge of the 'facts' – the search for some kind of infallible technical rule shows no sign of abating. The current craze, of course, is to supplant moral values by economic ones.

The result of this and other such attempts is always the same: the force of what is essentially moral judgment becomes attached to what purports to be a merely technical or dispassionately 'scientific' judgment, so that the latter comes to be asserted with a strangely puzzling ferocity. Michael Polanyi* called this process 'moral inversion'. In the case of apologists for the operations of 'the market' this kind of moral ferocity is unmistakable, and Adam Smith's 'invisible hand' becomes tacitly invested with positively awesome authority, while opponents of the system are attacked with all the vituperative fervour of religious bigotry.

Moral judgment and moral values cannot be avoided, but only inverted. The attempt to remove questions of ethical value from the public arena leaves a vacuum which is immediately filled by fiercely moralistic systems of prescription and control which assert a claim to absolute sovereignty even as they protest their 'freedom' from values.

That something is cheap, for example, or 'cost-effective' involves nothing more exciting than its monetary value, and certainly confers upon it no *moral* worth. But if we attempt to remove from the sphere in which costs are counted the *moral* judgment of whether or not we *should* count them, we leave a vacuum which is immediately filled by the inverted moral passion inhabiting, for example, the epithet 'effective' which seemed so innocently linked with 'cost'. Invertedly moral expressions have a secret power which to some extent accounts for their ferocity: we bury in the expression 'cost-effective' an assertion of moral superiority which is at the same time disclaimed and therefore cannot be submitted to ethical discussion. In fact, in supposedly making a purely 'scientific' economic judgment, we assert an invertedly moral judgment which,

*M. Polanyi, *Personal Knowledge*, Routledge and Kegan Paul, 1958.

simply because it is out of sight, makes it almost impossible for us to ask whether something is right just because it is cost-effective. All forms of discourse or rhetoric which purport to be 'value free' and yet which attempt to give direction to our lives are riddled with moralistic maxims disguised as matters of fact.

Human beings cannot escape moral judgment and ethical precept if only because they alone determine the ends of their own conduct. We are the subjects, not the objects of our world, and nothing (except, perhaps, the unexpected revelation of itself by a Supreme Being) could relieve us of the necessity for deciding what we do. Once power has become distributed unevenly within a society, however, it is in the interests of those with more, to hide from those who have less both the universality of the application of moral standards and the inevitability of moral action as the way of making the future. The inversion of moral values, and the discrediting of ethical conduct as somehow 'unscientific' both have the merit, from a viewpoint towards the top of the power hierarchy, of furthering the idea that our social order is based upon natural rather than man-made laws: inequality, injustice and exploitation thus become the natural order of things rather than issues which could or should be open to moral questioning and debate.

The airing in public of issues having a high moral content, except at carefully prescribed times and places, comes to be associated with disreputability or bad taste. The discussion of 'politics or religion', for example, is almost proverbially seen as something bordering on the indecent if performed outside those arenas specially constructed to contain it. The 'privatization' of ethical considerations not only removes them from the public sphere in which they may challenge established forms of exploitation, but also renders them more amenable to manipulation. Mystification in this respect is quickly achieved: it is hard for us now to see why men of good will in the eighteenth century were outraged by the idea of the secret ballot as a way of voting on matters of political importance. However, a little reflection suggests easily enough how secrecy in this respect, while purporting to allow people's political will to operate in unmolested privacy, actually makes it more possible to manipulate their conduct through underhand appeals to their interest. The slightly furtive atmosphere of the voting booth is thus by no means an entirely accidental phenomenon, but reflects the extent to which public courage and candour in discussing and contributing to policies which determine the nature of our communal life have been transformed into an officially sanctioned reticence about what we stand for and why. We discharge our public duty, or such remnants of it as are left, in silence and secrecy in a solitary act of political consummation once every four or five years.

The attachment of shame to public passion in matters of moral debate is but another way of maintaining discipline without the use of force at the same time as permitting the networks of interest to proliferate unchallenged. At the time when Kant wrote his *Critique of Practical Reason* it was still possible to regard the airing of ethical questions in public as one of the noblest activities in which people could engage, and he leaves us in no doubt either as to the error of confusing moral principles with considerations of interest. Since this was close to the time when the 'pursuit of happiness' was being written into the American Declaration of Independence and the British Utilitarians were busily trying to construct a calculus of happiness with which to solve the problem of moral uncertainty, Kant presumably had a clear sight of what was afoot. In formulating his 'categorical imperative' ('So act that the maxim of your will could always hold at the same time as a principle establishing universal law') Kant is at pains to show that, since one person's happiness is not necessarily linked with that of others, happiness cannot rationally be pursued without transgressing the fundamental moral rule that you should do as you would be done by. Though his language is a little awkward on modern ears, his contempt for the pursuit of happiness is plain:

> Now, if I say that my will is subject to a practical law, I cannot put forward my inclination ([e.g.] my avarice) as fit to be a determining ground of a universal practical law. It is so far from being worthy of universal legislation that in the form of a universal law it must destroy itself.
>
> It is therefore astonishing how intelligent men have thought of proclaiming as a universal practical law the desire for happiness, and therewith to make this desire the determining ground of the will merely because this desire is universal. Though elsewhere natural laws make everything harmonious, if one here attributed the universality of law to this maxim, there would be the extreme opposite of harmony, the most arrant conflict, and the complete annihilation of the maxim itself and its purpose. For the wills of all do not have one and the same object, but each person has his own (his own welfare), which, to be sure, can accidentally agree with the purposes of others who are pursuing their own, though this agreement is far from sufficing for a law because the occasional exceptions which one is permitted to make are endless and cannot be definitely comprehended in a universal rule.

It is moving now to encounter in his text Kant's uncomplicated faith in reason and his commitment to a social community in which it seemed axiomatic that others should be valued as the self. But while he puts to shame those professional apologists for the market economy some of whom pass for moral and political philosophers these days, we have nevertheless become so saturated in and hardened to the values and rhetoric of interest that it is almost impossible to share with Kant the inarticulate premises of his argument – he takes for granted a moral sentiment in the reader which today has all but disappeared from view.

Its disappearance from view does however not entail a diminution of its force – as I have tried to show, inverted moral passion becomes attached to statements of 'scientific fact' or to moralistic exhortations to others to conform to standards which are taken as indisputably valid, and comes to be used as a kind of, literally, secret weapon with which to bludgeon doubters. But it *is* always possible to ask of 'indisputable' standards, and indeed of any prescription masquerading as fact, whether it is good or right and whether we ought to obey it. These are questions we cannot escape because it is inconceivable that any authority other than our own will ever be established to guide our conduct, and even the fact that our moral decisions could in theory be shown by an (again inconceivable) objective observer to be determined by our history and experience, does not relieve us from the necessity of making them. It is an absolutely inescapable necessity of human existence that we assign value to our conduct.

For this reason, the ways in which society is ordered must always be open to ethical questioning, and all attempts (guided by interest) to associate the social order with some kind of impersonal necessity or authority are bound to be mystifications aimed at obscuring from people their freedom to challenge the *status quo* on moral grounds. While the pursuit of private happiness has become the obsession of our age, the possibility of 'public happiness' – the opportunity to engage publicly in the discussion, determination and implementation of value – has become eroded to the point of disappearance, and an apparatus for involvement in public affairs is excluded and prevented by an apparatus of discipline. Ethical instruction and discussion has become a purely private and informal matter unsupported by any institution of public life, and indeed for most people does not take place at all in any organized way. Even the churches, though of course always deriving ethical guidance from an essentially magical authority, have now more or less entirely abandoned moral teaching in favour of a euphoric commodification of magico-religious and deeply irrational 'goods' supposed to protect 'Christians' from the brutalities of this world and provide them with spiritual satisfactions barely distinguishable from the gratifications we are led to expect from the purchase of consumer durables.

The inescapable facts of existence – the exigencies of being embodied in time and space – mean that there is no possibility that the process whereby we assign value to conduct will disappear (and indeed without an at least tacit sense of right and wrong one could not act at all), but our articulation of this process and our development and institutionalization of an explicit understanding of it may well do so. If our interests, particularly in the shape of greed, exploitation and mindless damage, are not to run riot completely unchecked, we are going rapidly to have to recollect and recover our ability to submit them to ethical criticism and to repudiate any sense of intellectual disreputability or even shame which may, through the structures of interest, come to be attached to our endeavour. This task is appallingly difficult, since it will have to be done without the help of God, indeed without the help of any objective authority at all, and in the face of the concerted opposition of all those who, knowingly or unknowingly, stand to gain from the inequalities of our hierarchy of power (not to mention those who *think* they gain from what they believe to be the best of all possible worlds).

Because much of our conduct is inevitably enacted towards an open and evolving world, there is no possibility that we can settle upon a kind of permanently enshrined code of ethics, and the content of our moral prescriptions need be no more stable than our judgment of truth (the degree of accuracy of 'factual' statements changes constantly over time even though at any one point we are, not unreasonably, quite ready to say what 'the truth' of a given question is). This suggests that, for example, Kant's attempt to identify the *form* of moral precepts is much better founded than attempts to decide, in any absolute sense, upon their content. But there are in any case some chracteristics of ethical conduct which do not seem reasonably disputable, and one is the likelihood that observance of moral principle will often operate against individual interest. Treating others as one would wish to be treated oneself means that on occasion, indeed perhaps frequently, one will have for the sake of others to forego pleasures or advantages which would otherwise be quite easily obtained. Unless one defines 'interest' so widely as to make self-indulgence synonymous with altruism, then, what is in one's interest is often likely to conflict with what is right, and in fact one might almost say that such conflict is a *mark* of moral conduct.

It seems altogether likely that human societies are unable to organize themselves without a degree of inequality, and that, therefore, disparities in power are inevitable. The ideal of a just and equal society in which care is taken that every member of it shall be able to develop his or her potentialities to the full, and in which, for example, largely illusory processes of therapy are rendered unnecessary through the ministrations of love, represents an achievement so distant as to be indescribable in any coherent formulation. But this does not mean that we should attempt to make a virtue of necessity, or even take advantage of our plight, by arguing that we should morally endorse forms of social organization which we can see no way of changing. It is precisely the function of an ethics to combat and contain forms of conduct envisaged as ineradicable. Were sin easily banished, merely a technical imperfection on the face of the social world, there would be no need for morality.

What is so disturbing, if also so inevitable, about the structure of interest, is that it equates moral value with an assertion of its own aims. Such an equation is already apparent in embryo in the formulations of 'enlightened self-interest' of the Utilitarian philosophers of the eighteenth century, though they would no doubt have been horrified to see where their arguments would lead. Today, the 'freedom to choose' on the basis of an accepted and unquestioned inequality already built into the social structure, the valuation of appearances and 'public relations' above respect for embodied actuality, and the translation of exploitation into appeals to the virtuousness of 'giving people what they want', suggest an almost total submergence of morality in interest.

Most of the evils of our society, and certainly by far the greater part of the so-called 'pathological' emotional distress experienced by its members, are more or less directly attributable to the unequal distribution of forms of (usually economic) power which are abused and corrupting. Up until very recently even those maximally benefiting from the abuse of power and maximally corrupted by it would at least have paid lip-service to the view that such abuse was wrong, and, even if hypocritically, would have been able to make a conceptual distinction between morality and interest. The time is now fast arriving when to make such distinctions is seen simply as 'wet', and before long it may become almost impossible for 'ordinary people' to make it at all; already it has become virtually impossible for many people to see beyond a blinkered interest-stratum in the power hierarchy, and even in my personal experience I have come across many situations in which people are unable to conceive that economic considerations – for example questions of 'efficiency and effectiveness' in the running of the British National Health Service – do not coincide exactly with moral questions of right and wrong.

And yet, if one is to be able to understand the processes whereby people become unable to realize their potentialities in public living, to learn how to make a bodily contribution to the social world, to treat each other with kindness and forbearance as ends rather than means, and to become, as it were, the organic custodians of an unknowable future, the ability ethically to criticize the social structures in which we live is one which will have actively to be preserved. Not, of course, that the ability to make moral judgments will of itself change the world, but it is certainly a prerequisite to the kind of moral and political action by which the actual structures and institutions of society may be altered. The ills we suffer are not consequent upon our personal inadequacies or moralistically attributed faults: they are the inevitable result of publicly endorsed and communally practised forms of indifference, greed and exploitation, and require a moral reformation of our public, not our private ways of life. Instead of abusing power, we need to use whatever power we have to increase the power of others, to take care rather than treat, to enlighten rather than mystify, to love rather than exploit, and, in general, to think seriously about what are the obligations as opposed to the advantages of power. Ideally, the foremost obligation on power is to 'deconstruct' itself.

All this, no doubt, is hopelessly idealistic, and it is salutary to remember that, even were they possible, changes of heart would have little impact on the real world unless accompanied by highly organized and concerted action. However, an impotent recognition of moral failure is in my view preferable to a misguided trust in technical solutions which simply serve to justify further abuses. It is in any case difficult to be optimistic about the future: perhaps the only way the social world evolves is by lurching forward through revolution and catastrophe.

It is difficult enough – indeed bordering on the impossible – for individuals to mend their ways following therapeutic insight; how societies do it (unless, indeed, through the shedding of blood or the making of catastrophic mistakes) is infinitely more difficult to see. But unless our society *does* mend its ways we may expect no improvement to occur in our private lives, no greater satisfaction in 'relationships'; there will be no 'breakthroughs' in scientific or psychological understanding to patch up our unhappiness and allow us to carry on as before.

In trying to think about the future, it may be instructive to consider for a moment a more or less random selection of the views of some of those whose thought has contributed to these pages. All of them are people who were deeply critical of the economic and political structures in which they found themselves, in some cases making just about the blackest possible diagnosis of the social ills of their time, and yet all of them also orientate themselves to the future with optimism.

Particularly poignant is the view expressed by William Godwin, the Utilitarian political philosopher whose *Enquiry Concerning Political Justice*, published in 1793, is taken by many as one of the principle intellectual foundations upon which to build opposition to governmental power and its abuse:

> Wealth was at one period almost the single object of pursuit that presented itself to the gross and uncultivated mind. Various objects will hereafter divide men's attention, the love of liberty, the love of equality, the pursuits of art and the desire of knowledge. These objects will not, as now, be confined to a few, but will gradually be laid open to all. The love of liberty obviously leads to a sentiment of union, and a disposition to sympathize in the concerns of others. The general diffusion of truth will be productive of general improvement; and men will daily approximate towards those views according to which every object will be appreciated at its true value. Add to which, that the improvement of which we speak is public, and not individual. The progress is the progress of all. Each man will find his sentiments of justice and rectitude echoed by the sentiments of his neighbours. Apostasy will be made eminently improbable, because the apostate will incur, not only his own censure, but the censure of every beholder.

A century later, Leo Tolstoy, who spent the second half of his life close to despair over the state of society but whose world-wide influence and fame as a moral thinker is now largely forgotten, wrote the following:

> 'One trembles before the present horrible condition of human life: taxes, clergy, great landed properties, prisons, guillotines, cannon, dynamite, millionaires and beggars. In reality all these horrors are the result of our own acts. Not only can they disappear, but they must disappear, in conformity with the new conscience of humanity. Christ said that He had conquered the world; and in fact He has conquered it. Dreadful as it may be, the evil no longer really exists because it is disappearing from the consciences of men.
>
> 'Today humanity is passing through a transitory phase. Everything is ready for passing from one state of the human condition to another; it needs only a slight push to set it off and it can take place at any minute.
>
> 'The social conscience of humanity already condemns the

former way of life and is ready to adopt the new. The whole world feels it, and is convinced of it. But inertia and fear of the unknown retards the application in practice of what has for a long time been realized in theory. In such cases it sometimes needs only one word to make the force called public opinion change the whole order of things at once, and do it without struggle or violence.

'The freeing of men from servitude, from ignorance, can not be obtained by revolution, syndicates, peace congresses, etc., but simply by the conscience of each one of us forbidding us to participate in violence and asking us in amazement: Why are you doing that?

'It is enough for us to emerge from the hypnosis that hides our true mission from us, for us to ask with dread and indignation how any one can insist upon our committing such horrible crimes. And this awakening can take place at any instant.'

This is what I wrote fifteen years ago, and I repeat today with conviction that this awakening is about to take place.

Certainly I shall not be there to take part in it, I, an old man, more than eighty years of age; but I know with the same certainty as I see spring follow winter and night day, that this hour has already come in the life of Christian humanity.*

In 1921 R. H. Tawney's *The Acquisitive Society* was published. In its final paragraph Tawney states its principal conclusions and predicts the disappearance from society of purely economic preoccupations with a confidence beginning to sound rather familiar:

The burden of our civilization is not merely, as many suppose, that the product of industry is ill-distributed, or its conduct tyrannical, or its operation interrupted by embittered disagreements. It is that industry itself has come to hold a position of exclusive predominance among human interests, which no single interest, and least of all the provision of the material means of existence, is fit to occupy. Like a hypochondriac who is so absorbed in the processes of his own digestion that he goes to his grave before he has begun to live, industrialized communities neglect the very objects for which it is worth while to acquire riches in their feverish preoccupation with the means by which riches can be acquired.

*L. Tolstoy, *The Law of Love and the Law of Violence*, Anthony Blond, 1970.

That obsession by economic issues is as local and transitory as it is repulsive and disturbing. To future generations it will appear as pitiable as the obsession of the seventeenth century by religious quarrels appears today; indeed, it is less rational, since the object with which it is concerned is less important. And it is a poison which inflames every wound and turns every trivial scratch into a malignant ulcer. Society will not solve the particular problems of industry which afflict it until that poison is expelled, and it has learned to see industry itself in the right perspective. If it is to do that, it must rearrange its scale of values. It must regard economic interests as one element in life, not as the whole of life. It must persuade its members to renounce the opportunity of gains which accrue without any corresponding service, because the struggle for them keeps the whole community in a fever. It must so organize its industry that the instrumental character of economic activity is emphasized by its subordination to the social purpose for which it is carried on.

Many of those writing in more recent times, particularly perhaps in the United States, tend to combine the bleakest views of the past and present with an optimistic trust in youth to put matters right. Paul Goodman, for example, saw in the attitudes of the 'beat generation' and the 'angry young men' of the 1950s hope that the tide might be turning:

I think that the existential reality of Beat, Angry, and Delinquent behaviour is indicated by the fact that other, earnest, young fellows who are not themselves disaffected and who are not phony, are eager to hear about them, and respect them. One cannot visit a university without being asked a hundred questions about them.

Finally, some of these groups are achieving a simpler fraternity, animality, and sexuality than we have had, at least in America, in a long, long time.

This valuable program is in direct contrast to the mores of what we have in this book been calling 'the organized system', its role playing, its competitiveness, its canned culture, its public relations, and its avoidance of risk and self-exposure. That system and its mores are death to the spirit, and any rebellious group will naturally raise a contrasting banner.

Now the organized system is very powerful and in its full tide of success, apparently sweeping everything before it in science, education, community planning, labor, the arts, not to speak of business and politics where it is indigenous. Let me say that we of the previous generation who have been sickened and enraged to see earnest and honest effort and humane culture swamped by this muck, are heartened by the crazy young allies, and we think that perhaps the future may make more sense than we dared hope.*

Only a few years later Lewis Mumford's almost savagely revealing analysis of the evils wrought on society by the impersonal violence of a technology of power is unexpectedly and almost incongruously muted by views such as the following:

The yearning for a primitive counter-culture, defying the rigidly organized and depersonalized forms of Western civilization, began to float into the Western mind in the original expressions of Romanticism among the intellectual classes. That desire to return to a more primeval state took a folksy if less articulate form, in the elemental rhythms of jazz, more than half a century ago. What made this idea suddenly erupt again, with almost volcanic power, into Western society was its incarnation in the Beatles. It was not just the sudden success of the Beatles' musical records that indicated that a profound change was taking place in the minds of the young: it was their new personality, as expressed in their long, neo-mediaeval haircut, their unabashed sentimentality, their nonchalant posture, and their dreamlike spontaneity that opened up for the post-nuclear generation the possibility of an immediate escape from mega-technic society. In the Beatles all their repressions, and all their resentments of repression were released: by hairdo, costume, ritual, and song, all changes depending upon purely personal choice, the new counter-ideas that bound the younger generation together were at once clarified and magnified. Impulses that were still too dumbly felt for words, spread like wildfire through incarnation and imitation.†

What strikes a chill in the contemporary reader's heart about such passages as these (which fell easily to hand – I did not have to comb libraries to unearth them) is that their future has now come, and perhaps even gone, with none of the expected improvement. What possibilities Godwin saw in an understanding of the nature of 'happiness', his faith in the good will of those with the power to reason, have been mercilessly betrayed in the pursuit of interest. Tolstoy's intimation of a revival of Christian ethics would

---

*Growing Up Absurd, op. cit.
† L. Mumford, The Pentagon of Power, Secker and Warburg, 1971.

surely have been sadly extinguished by now. Tawney's was no doubt a longer view, but even in this case one wonders whether he would have been so sanguine could he have witnessed the speed with which the more caring society for which he worked so hard is currently being dismantled. And we have now had the chance to observe for ourselves the growing up of the beats, the angry young men and the Beatles: all securely locked within the deadly serious world of the market, privately preoccupied with success or survival, some dead and some assassinated.

So how to account for such optimism on the part of people whose gaze on their contemporary scene was so penetrating, so honest and so unflinching? Perhaps in part they were the victims of the mistaken belief that cure must follow an accurate diagnosis, perhaps they were misled by their passionate hope or by over-generalizing their own good will. Perhaps, again, it is impossible for humane men and women, however black the portents, to envisage the future with anything but at least a degree of optimism.

It is not at all difficult, certainly, to bring out the ostrich in those unable to contemplate without pain the ways we conduct ourselves towards each other. We can drop out into 'counter-cultures'; we can become 'born again' into the magical belief systems of fundamentalist religions. Perhaps, even, we really can create through science and technology a dream-world shaped entirely by our wishes and in which we could live our lives encapsulated in fantastic gratification. But in the end, I believe, none of these 'solutions' represents anything other than extremes of wishful thinking, a kind of communal madness from which embodied truth would one day drag us back to a devasted reality.

The development of 'counter-cultures' relying on some form of magical or ideological escape from the larger social world, simply evades the difficulties of getting to grips with the structures which cause us such distress. An entirely justified and understandable disgust with the abuse of scientific knowledge and technological power leads to the wishful positing of alternatives which side-step experience and challenge rationality. While welcoming and endorsing much of the theory and practice of what he calls the 'party of Narcissus' – i.e. of those aligning themselves with feminism, environmentalism and the peace movement, etc. – Christopher Lasch takes a line very similar to that argued in this book:

> It is the deterioration of public life, together with the privatiz-ation and trivialization of moral ideas, that prevents a collab-orative assault on the environmental and military difficulties confronting modern nations. But the party of Narcissus does not understand the source of these difficulties: the confusion

of practice with technique. It shares this confusion and thus repudiates all forms of purposeful action in favor of playful, artistic pursuits, which it misunderstands, moreover, as activities without structure or purpose. When it insists on the pathology of purposefulness, it merely reverses industrial ideology. Where the prevailing ideology swallows up practice into a cult of technique, the 'counterculture' indiscriminately rejects both and advocates a renunciation of will and purpose as the only escape from Promethean technology. Disparaging human inventiveness, which it associates only with destructive industrial technologies, it defines the overriding imperative of the present age as a return to nature. It ignores the more important need to restore the intermediate world of practical activity, which binds man to nature in the capacity of a loving caretaker and cultivator, not in a symbiotic union that simply denies the reality of man's separation from nature.*

In the last few paragraphs of his sweeping and deeply impressive three-volume historical analysis of the economic structures of the modern world, Fernand Braudel perhaps comes closer than anyone to giving us a glimpse of what we are up against:

Jean-Paul Sartre may have dreamed of a society from which inequality would have disappeared, where one man would not exploit another. But no society in the world has yet given up tradition and the use of privilege. If this is ever to be achieved, all the social hierarchies will have to be overthrown, not merely those of money or state power, not only social privilege but the uneven weight of the past and of culture. The experience of the socialist countries proves that the disappearance of a single hierarchy — the economic hierarchy — raises scores of new problems and is not enough on its own to establish equality, liberty or even plenty. A clear-sighted revolution, if such a thing is even possible — and if it were, would the paralysing weight of circumstances allow it to remain so for long? — would find it very difficult to demolish what should be demolished, while retaining what should be retained: freedom for ordinary people, cultural independence, a market economy with no loaded dice, and a little fraternity. It is a very tall order — especially since whenever capitalism is challenged, it is invariably during a period of economic difficulty, whereas far-reaching structural reform, which

*The Minimal Self, op. cit.

would inevitably be difficult and traumatic, requires a context of abundance or even superabundance. And the present population explosion is likely to do little or nothing to encourage the more equitable distribution of surpluses.*

The conclusion to Braudel's gargantuan intellectual undertaking, though stated undramatically enough, strikes, especially in the light of others' optimism, an unusually sombre note:

> If people set about looking for them, seriously and honestly, economic solutions could be found which would extend the area of the market and would put at its disposal the economic advantages so far kept to itself by one dominant group in society. But the problem does not essentially lie there; it is social in nature. Just as a country at the centre of a world-economy can hardly be expected to give up its privileges at international level, how can one hope that the dominant groups who combine capital and state power, and who are assured of international support, will agree to play the game and hand over to someone else?

Can one then really not *hope* that people will act against their own immediate interests? Either the question as posed by Braudel is a rhetorical statement of despair, or it demands an answer.

Hope is a very private matter, and what grounds for hope I may find in my own experience are therefore likely to be of little use to anyone else. However, perhaps there are some observations which may be found sustaining. One – the most important – is that people uncorrupted by power and unblinded by interest (and therefore most often to be found at the very base of the social hierarchy) are in my experience perfectly able and often eager to act lovingly and altruistically when permitted (which is rare) the space to do so. It seems to me, again, that reflection able to break free from injunctions to the pursuit of happiness quite quickly suggests that the only life worth living is one which points beyond itself. And from the perspective of history the past is short and the future long; we have yet to try living by an ethics which is based neither on God nor on slavery.

From the point of view of public life, however, there are altogether cooler and more rational reasons for conducting ourselves *as if* hope for the future were justified. Not the least of these is that, even though we may be sure that they will involve us in the greatest

---

*F. Braudel, *Civilization and Capitalism 15th–18th Century*, 3 vols., Fontana, 1985.

difficulty, we cannot possibly foretell what our endeavours may lead to.

It may indeed be impossible from our present position to envisage a society in which the hierarchies of which Braudel writes could be dismantled, but though the weight of the evidence which he reviews is almost crushingly dismaying, the span of history is still extremely short. What lends a note almost of fatuity to some of the more optimistic prognostications quoted above is the *immediacy* of the improvement they envisage. Having correctly identified the grave shortcomings of a society which pursues instant happiness, they then themselves propose an instant remedy for them. The absence of an instant remedy, however, the impossibility of the 'cure' we all – as I have argued, misguidedly – so readily seek also for our personal distress, is not a reason for resigned acceptance of the inevitability of exploitation and greed and the harm they do. What we need, rather, is to develop the very seriousness and honesty which Braudel acknowledges as possible, to foster a patient 'care-fulness' designed to last over generations, and to recognize that greed and exploitation, even if they cannot be wiped out within any imaginable span of time, must be opposed. It is precisely the possibilities for the development of any such opposition which have become so drastically eroded in recent times by interests which have the power to collapse the kind of moral space in which they *can* develop.

The privatization and inversion of the moral impulse of 'ordinary people' impose upon them a moralism which asserts that not only are their difficulties and distress their 'own fault', but that the remedy also is somehow up to them as private individuals. Moral responsibility, which should be *socially recognized* as an integral part of an individual's public duty, thus becomes a kind of private burden, and the onus for changing the world falls with a punitive heaviness on each one of us as something we have to wrestle with on our own. Now there is of course a perfectly acceptable sense in which 'things will only change' through the separate contributions of individual embodied subjects, but in saying this it is easy to overlook the fact that a person cannot act at all unless he or she has the space in which to do so.

There are very many people, worried and concerned about the state of the world and of society, whose moral integrity and fortitude lead them to accept with resignation that 'you can only do what you can'. In this, they are rather like those 'patients' not infrequently encountered in psychotherapy who accept that 'there's only me who can do anything about it' and who struggle bravely against an often inimical world. But though there is certainly truth in this attitude as far as it goes, it overlooks a dimension absolutely essential to the effectiveness of action, i.e. the public dimension which combines with private intention or impulse to open up a moral space.

In order to change things for the better — in order, that is, to be able to *act* morally — the individual must have the moral *space* in which to do so. This is not something which people can create for themselves as private individuals, but something which is socially created and maintained through the proper use of concerted (political) power. A politics which perverts and abuses power in order to operate a network of vested interests collapses the space in which people can conduct themselves instrumentally to exercise a public function, and it does this mainly by focusing attention on purely private needs and treating 'politically motivated' conduct as somehow suspect or reprehensible. If, however, we are to come to see that we are inflicting incurable but avoidable damage on each other rather than merely suffering personally unavoidable but curable 'breakdown', if, that is, we are to move from an ideology of therapy to a culture of care, we shall have to force open around ourselves a moral space which gives us room for concerted action, and this can only be done through the re-insertion into that space of a 'public dimension'. We shall have, to put it another way, to re-establish an ethical politics in the place of an apparatus of power for the manipulation of interest. It is important to remember, furthermore, that we need to do this not to change our *selves* nor to try magically to put right injuries irrevocably inflicted, but to set up a framework in which future injuries may perhaps be avoided.

It is simply too much to expect people to take on the moral burden of their own suffering, however much therapy we may offer them. Much of what people take to be their own private misery is generated within the social structure in which everyone is located, and is therefore, in every sense, a matter for the greatest public concern.

Index

Adler, A., 113
'Angry Young Men', 155, 157
Arendt, H., 30–1, 35
Ariès, P., 115n
astrology, 48–9

Bacon, F., 50
'Beat Generation', 155, 157
beauty, 141
behaviourism, 46, 51
Bion, W., 12, 13n
blame, 6, 66–72, 76, 90, 115, 145
bliss, memory of, 26–7, 33, 73,
    123–4
Boorstin, D., 10n
Braudel, F., 158–60
bulimia, 42
Buss, R., 65n

Calderón, P., 7
caring, 72
categorical imperative, 148
change, 44, 79–81, 84–7, 90–1
children, 106, 113–20, 127,
    135–6
Christianity, 138, 143
Church, the, 17, 29, 149
comfort, 4, 6, 46, 48, 51, 91, 142
commitment, 96, 107, 112
commodity, 19, 33, 93–4, 96–7,
    103–4
Comte, A., 18, 48
consumption, 39, 97, 117, 126,
    132
counter-culture, 157
cruelty, 120
culture, 19, 132–5, 138
cure, 15, 48, 73, 79–82, 85–6, 90,
    122

Danziger, K., 64, 65n
daughters, 106, 114–15

Davidson, N., 73n
death instinct, 28
Debord, G., 10n
delinquency, 54
demystification, 4–5
determinism, 75
Dickens, C., 20, 139
difficulty, 88, 91, 122, 128
discipline, 53–5, 67, 128–30, 142,
    148–9
disease, 73–4
disillusion, 109–10
divination, 48
Divoky, D., 53n, 55, 58
dreams, 2, 7–11, 16, 75, 81, 120,
    128, 140–1

embodiedness, 11, 13, 74–5, 120,
    133, 138–42
encounter groups, 99, 102
encouragement, 4–5, 48, 51, 126,
    142
Enlightenment, the, 29
equality, 77, 142
examinations, 54–5
'excellence', 136
exploitation, 69, 77, 89, 106, 115,
    120, 143, 147, 152, 160
Eysenck, H. J., 57

factory farming, 37, 87
faith, 132
familiarity, 34, 36, 89, 142
family, 106, 113–19
Farber, L. H., 75n
fathers, 106, 114–15
fault, 19, 67–8, 77, 109
feelings, 72–4, 127, 129
fixation, 126–8
Foucault, M., 53–5, 58, 65, 67,
    103, 113
freedom, 76, 91

163

Index